COVER ME

CLASS IN AMERICA

Series Editor
Jeffrey R. Di Leo

University of Nebraska Press | Lincoln and London

COVER ME

A HEALTH INSURANCE MEMOIR

SONYA HUBER

Acknowledgments for the use of
copyrighted material appear on
page x, which constitutes
an extension of the copyright page.

Library of Congress
Cataloging-in-Publication Data
Huber, Sonya, 1971–
Cover me: a health insurance memoir / Sonya Huber.
    p.   cm. — (Class in America)
ISBN 978-0-8032-2623-4 (cloth : alk. paper)
1. Huber, Sonya, 1971–
2. Medically uninsured women—
United States—Biography.
3. Columbus (Ohio)—Biography.
I. Title.
RA413.7.U53H83 2010
368.38′20092—dc22
[B]
2009050226

Set in Quadraat Sans by Bob Reitz.
Designed by R. W. Boeche.

To Peter Christopher, 1956–2008
To Ivan for every day

CONTENTS

ACKNOWLEDGMENTS

Thank you to my friends for their support and their willingness to have pieces of their stories told in this book, including Kathy Bohley, Ami Peacock, Jenny Grabmeier, Brooke Davis and Margaret Fox, Sharad Puri, Nicole Stellon O'Donnell, Monica Kieser, Arwen Wilder, and Steve Young. Thank you to my family, including my brother Glenn, my sister Nicole, and my parents, for their amazing tolerance and support through the bizarre experience of having a memoirist in the family. Thanks also to Skate in appreciation for the shared experiences in this book, and best wishes on your path. Thank you to my son Ivan for every single day of joy, for your sweetness and spirit and energy.

Thank you to the employers over the years who gave me benefits or who couldn't but wanted to, including Cathy Levine of UHCAN and my many employers at the Ohio State University. I am grateful for the guiding mentorship of Lee Martin and Bill Roorbach, two writers and friends who have never hesitated to share their wisdom and encouragement. Thank you to Bill and also to Sue William Silverman for vital feedback on an earlier draft of this manuscript; a sincere thank you to Ladette Randolph, former editor and interim director of the University of Nebraska Press, who found this book a home; thank you also to the talented staff of the University of Nebraska Press.

This book would not exist in its present form without Cliff Price's extensive advice and support. Cliff, thank you for your love, insight, encouragement, and steadying influence. Though you appear at the end of this work, you are never an afterthought; I am profoundly grateful for the new beginning I found at the end of this story.

This is a work of creative nonfiction and, as such, is an exploration into the limits of memory and the folly of the human heart. Narrative arcs appear on these pages where lived experience showed only confusion and fear. Mistakes abound; I tried my best; I take full responsibility for the errors contained in these pages. The names of a few people, such as Skate and J—— have been changed.

The author gratefully acknowledges the editors who published early chapters of this work as stand-alone essays. All work is reprinted here with permission.

Chapter 1 originally appeared as "Waiting for the Placebo Effect" in *Clapboard House*, Spring 2009.

Chapter 3 originally appeared as "Anointing of the Sick" in *Hotel Amerika*, Spring 2008.

Chapter 5 originally appeared in a slightly different form as "Female Trouble" in the *Oxford Magazine* 22 (Summer 2008).

Chapter 7 originally appeared as "Prescriptions" in *Sweet: A Literary Confection* 1, no. 2 (Spring 2009).

Chapter 8 originally appeared in a slightly different form as "Employee + Child(ren)" in the *Washington Post Magazine*, August 3, 2008.

WAITING FOR THE PLACEBO EFFECT

My sinuses throbbed and pressed against the bones of my face like overcooked bratwurst. I pulled open the glass door of the community co-op in Columbus, Ohio. I wanted to fill my skull with brightly colored vitamin cocaine and blot out the suicide gray midwestern sky.

Yes, I should probably have been sitting in a doctor's office.

I was an adjunct teaching writing at a local university. I was uninsured—or so I thought, but that's another story. The Human Resources lady didn't even mention health insurance during our two-minute tax form session that fall of 2004. No benefits packet arrived in my mailbox, so I assumed I was in the lecturer job class with all the other guns for hire on campus. My husband, a self-employed carpenter whom I'll call Skate, fixed his swollen thumbs by drilling holes in his fingernails to let out the pus. We were do-it-yourselfers of the involuntary variety.

I spent my days swilling coffee, wincing at the onslaught of traffic and lateness and e-mails. I ate Sudafed like cinnamon red hots. As if my South Side of Chicago accent wasn't nasal enough (Chicauuuuugo), I honked with the voice-squeezing pressure of the constantly congested.

I wanted to lie down on the brownish gray carpet and wait for a

vegan staffer to drag me into the break room and heal me with cam-
phor-and-echinacea steam and homeopathic herbal tinctures.

Insurance was invented for ship captains in the 1660s who needed
protection from the risks of the frothing, pounding sea. Once insured,
these seamen could leave their wrecked vessels to founder on the
rocks. Insurance was described in 1665 as "[t]he Covenant of pre-
venting Danger . . . [which] added a Shadow of Law; whereby the
incertainty of the Event is usually transferred to another, with some
certain Reward."

The only reward I wanted was the safety that was so near and just
out of reach. It seemed to circle, to splash and taunt me, in whalelike
SUVs that circled the perimeter beltway of I-270, each shiny vehicle filled
with moms and kids who clearly did not worry about medical bills.

In those months, I drove the snow-sludged highways toward the
babysitters or job number one or job number three, all freelance gigs
without benefits. In a boil and fester of envy, I hated the SUVs and
their drivers because each of those people was *covered* and therefore
safe. They lived in another universe, where bodies and treatments
paired and came together effortlessly like ballroom dancers in layers of chiffon and satin.

I didn't want their cash. I had enough. I paid for coffees with my
girlfriends; dropped an occasional $15 for a sexy shirt on sale at Urban
Outfitters; and had enough pocket change for books, garage-sale
clogs, and thrift-store sweaters, for movies and sushi and Indian
food and all the other markers of comfort for a midwestern white
girl with a few master's degrees. I had credit card balances and
debt, yet I was also highly attuned to the aesthetics of a nice shoe.
The skim latte cup was either half empty or half full. I didn't want
cash; I wanted coverage.

In the co-op on that fevered and shivery day in early 2005, I locked
eyes with an Odwalla C-Monster Fruit Smoothie with 1,000 percent

the recommended daily allowance of vitamin C. I'm sure you have seen them: about four bucks for four mouthfuls of superhealthy puree (with profits heading straight to its parent company, Coca-Cola). Anyone who shells out cash for that scam has only herself to blame.

The plastic bottle of juice stood with its cousins, shoulder to shoulder, all colors of a tropical Gauguin painting of Tahiti, in a low cooler near a tall shelf of ground yarrow root and feverfew. Cheaper juices stood in uneven rows, their dusty glass surfaces adhered with stickers, $2.00 each, offering the exact same nutrients and vitamins. The cheap juices wore labels that were slightly less pretty, the ad copy slightly more modest and realistic.

In a magazine rack at the front of the co-op, near the cash register, my safe and successful alter ego cavorted in ads for Green Investment and ecotourism on the pages of the *Utne Reader*. She was a writer in Seattle or Santa Cruz, pulling her Aveda-scented hair into a ponytail, shrugging off her name-brand polar fleece, and then chugging a $3.99 Odwalla Smoothie as she piloted her new hybrid Prius on the way to a three-day yoga retreat.

I didn't want to be her.

Oh, shut up. Of course I did. I wanted to flaunt to the world, to imply with my Aveda-smelling skin and my woven fair-trade handbag that I had the embrace of Jesus and Buddha, the salvation security. I wanted to show the world the clear skin and steady gaze that come from nights of easy sleep, organic vegetables, and lack of stress.

What was going on in that Odwalla moment?

Ad copy ropes in an otherwise mostly sane woman; nothing unusual there. I'm not saying I'm particularly sane; I regularly spent the diaper money on spurious *Glamour* magazines and chocolate bars while my superego looked the other way.

But this was something different, a low point for me in which specific irrational costs and benefits tipped the scales toward Odwalla. Granted, I remember that day partially because the hippie universe delivered a left hook before I would even finish drinking that bottle of juice. But I'll get to that.

What I see there, looking at that woman standing in front of the cooler, is healthcare fatigue. I see a woman who wanted an Odwalla bedtime story of comfort, the same safety I exuded to my baby son when I read him *Snuggle Puppy* for the three trillionth time. I wanted to hear that the flannelled low-income princess could afford to make herself healthy.

I clearly could not. An office visit and prescription for my sinus infection would have set me back $100.

Maybe, instead, four bucks would work.

What I needed was the curative and sustaining break from sanity. I needed three minutes, eight swallows or so, in which simple faith would grant me the illusion that my actions mattered, that my own body was under my control.

By age thirty-three I had yelled into a megaphone for universal healthcare on the steps of the Ohio statehouse. I had enrolled my baby son in the state program for low-income families. I had seen my picture in the newspaper and heard my voice on the radio yelling about healthcare.

By age thirty-three I had already been sent to collections several times for medical debt. I worried about money, which sent cortisol and other stress hormones coursing through my body, triggering the fight-or-flight response that proclaimed an emergency and then subtly wore me down with the effort of staying on physical alert.

By age thirty-three I had lived through eleven gaps in healthcare coverage. During each, I wore a groove of worry in my frontal lobe that seemed directly connected to my lymph nodes, white blood cells, and serotonin levels. I want to know what life would have looked like without that undercurrent of healthcare anxiety and longing. I want to see a version of myself, body and mind, without that skein of tension.

Most of my friends cycled in and out of the same circus. The drunks told each other that beer sterilized your throat when you had a cold. The hipsters, who had formerly spent their time bitching about how punk was not dead, developed secondary specializations in acupuncture, green algae pills, craniosacral massage, wildflower homeopathic tinctures, Reiki, Chinese medicine, and various other non-Western therapies.

I'd already done Catholicism and considered my debt to hocus-pocus to have been paid. At that time in my life, I was able to finally hear the word "chakra" without throwing up, but I harbored a lingering distrust of New Agey thinking. But I also wondered if maybe my hipster-cum-hippie friends had it right. They could take back a portion of control over their bodies. Instead of worrying, maybe I should have been romancing my adrenal and lymph systems, cooking organic stir-fry, and meditating placidly while holding my sleeping infant son.

Drumming circles aside, the hippie culture of green algae pills and I had come to a sort of détente, because it seemed that receiving a squirt of herbal Rescue Remedy under the tongue took less time than whispering an extra Hail Mary. Like a doubting Catholic who goes to confession just in case, I shrugged and accepted anything that might conceivably work, including the placebo effect.

Nobody wanted to toss a barstool in rage at the cost of an ER visit or launch a punk-rock throwdown about an uninsured root canal. My women friends bitched about their boyfriends over coffee but didn't dredge up meaty curses toward their health plans. Fixing healthcare was more hopeless and pointless than waiting for the addict to stop drugging, than getting your brother to pay you the $300 he owed you, than waiting for your favorite band to get back together. Forget it. There's always bankruptcy.

I cradled the juice in my sweaty hand, pushing a hank of long brown hair behind my ear. My glasses were probably fogged up with the transition from the gray, wet cold outside to the steamy warmth of the co-op. I sniffed. I was tired, sick of carrying shredded coupons in my coat pockets. Sick of looking for the cheapest toilet paper. Sick of holding up the grocery lines with my WIC coupons while the cashier rolled her eyes and the people behind me looked me up and down. I hated the bleak cast that had settled over life itself for its potential expense. Every slip and fall, every cough, glinted with the knife-edge threat of a serious condition, a hospital visit, a debt of several thousand dollars I couldn't repay.

Some weakness—a fever surge or a howl of wind outside or a sinus pang—decided it.

Fuck it. Come here, sweet immunity sports car fantasy of life as ad copy. I ripped open the plastic seal and swigged the expensive juice.

The cool, sweet liquid splashed down my throat. Its thick texture felt healthy and substantial, as if it could flow to a fever-thinned weak spot and fill it like vitamin spackle. I lobbed my desperation toward the icons I worshipped, like lighting a novena candle in front of a Virgin Mary statue. As if by throwing money—$3.99 plus tax—toward a remote representative of my healthcare deity I could curry favor.

This is the story of my torrid and twisted love affair with health insurance.

I had known its embrace. Each blissful fling unfolded with delicious expectation, wet with whispers of forevermore. I entered these brief affairs with pink hope and the best of intentions. New health insurance cards—coy valentines—always arrived in plain white envelopes. Each plastic card was like a hotel room key that unlocked its own universe of safety and security, each with its own rules. Savoring my good fortune, I browsed the provider listing and chose a fresh crew of doctors to peer into my orifices. The courting and flirting began with a bit of game playing, the waiting periods and the occasional denial of coverage for preexisting conditions. After new love's rush of anticipation and insecurity, I made myself at home in each network, scattering the fragments of my medical history behind me like a trail of crushed candy hearts.

Take me. I'm yours. Hold me and never let me go.

I graduated from college in 1993 and leapt from the shelter of my parents' healthcare plan. The next fifteen years earned me a scattershot range of paychecks at twenty-five jobs. I was a receptionist many times over, a mental health counselor, a proofreader, writer, editor, reporter, assistant publisher, bookstore clerk, writing teacher, and community organizer. Eight of these gigs came with health insurance, and I latched on to those eight health plans with a desperation the employers often didn't deserve. I backed myself into gray partitioned cubicles to get screwed by boring, dead-end, or degrading jobs, faking enthusiasm all the way for the healthcare payoff.

In between my months of insurance, I gravitated toward loser, slacker, emotionally unavailable jobs that wouldn't support my healthcare needs. I've always had a thing for the bad boys, and maybe I kept unconsciously choosing those chain-walleted, tattooed health plans that looked fine in the dim and smoky light of a fling. The second my body exhibited a need, however, these health plans turned grouchy and distant, coughing up loopholes and denials of coverage. Maybe my full-coverage, low-deductible dreamboat was still out there somewhere, bobbing above the surface of the ocean as I muttered, "plenty of fish," and sorted the bottom-feeders below.

My healthcare hookup story is remarkable only in its mediocrity. I tried so hard to find the One and to discern the Rules. I hated the anonymous tryst of an emergency room visit, the feeling of a stranger's hands on my body and the knowledge that his parting words of "good luck" would be the last I'd hear from him. I wanted a Prince Charming—a general care practitioner, a personal care physician, a referring physician—to arrive with a fistful of referral slips. I wanted to go to an HMO where everybody knew my name.

Taking another sip, I stood in line at the register. When I got to the front, I presented my co-op membership card and paid the four bucks and change, signifying to myself that I was on the side of the healthy and those destined for health. I could fake it and pretend I was in a land where $3.99 was not that big of a deal. And somehow, this juice, this brief respite from penny pinching, unknotted my shoulders and my chest. The juice tasted lovely, sweet and tang whirled with a slight grit.

We can't always be hard, I was saying to myself, and that is also okay. Poor can't always mean the cheap juice. Crisis addressed, I swirled some juice around my teeth, sipped something complicated about my own weakness and my own need to acknowledge it off and on. I wavered in overlaps between the woozy shame of a needless purchase and the shrug of water or smoothie under the bridge. Fevers would pass.

I wanted to finish the juice inside in the warm co-op before buttoning my coat and heading out, chin tucked into my collar, into the whipping wind. I crumpled the receipt into my pocket and walked from the cash register toward the co-op bulletin board on the front wall. The bulletin board was covered with colored paper—hand-drawn ads promoting eco-friendly house cleaning, tantric pet minding, and a workshop for learning how to build your own herb garden.

Then I saw it: a flyer for an upcoming seminar, "Living Serenely without Health Insurance."

Serenely. Mango-berry puree pooled beneath my tongue as my bloodstream flushed with adrenaline. I stared at the flyer, riveted. I had never entertained the vile union of these two concepts: serenity and being uninsured.

I respect people who can talk about having gratitude for their addictions, who feel blessed by their cancers, and the like. But I am not yet on that spiritual plane. I am clearly somewhere far beneath it, in an underground foxhole of healthcare. I had to force myself to take in a breath. Maybe it was the fever, but I felt attacked by that innocent poster, which seemed to be calling me out as the spiritual midget I am.

The truth was that I wanted more than anything else to live serenely without health insurance, but I wasn't sure if that fantasy was akin to "peace within domestic violence" or "finding your pocket of calm in racial apartheid." Those pairings and strategies—strangely, profanely—are necessary to survive and yet evil to contemplate.

I wrapped my coat around me, shoved my orange knit ski cap on my head, and pushed open the glass door against the wind, gripping a half-empty bottle of juice that had lost its magic. I found my slush-encrusted car and blasted the defroster, watching the windshield wipers grate over hunks of ice on the windshield. I probably took off my glasses and cried, head down on the steering wheel, fever flushed.

I probably fumbled with my metal-cold cell phone and called my friend Kathy, a divorced single mom living with her two kids in her parents' basement. We laughed at each other's bad days, not unkindly, because we seemed to trade the same day back and forth as we traded tips about where to apply for low-income childcare and moaned about picking up bulk quantities of peanut butter from the WIC (Women, Infants, and Children) office.

"Oh, honey," she might have said. "Sounds like you need the Open."

The Open was a scrolled, two-inch, cast-iron fob that probably once hung in a store window. I don't know where it came from or who owned it first, but over the years of our friendship it had somehow become our Buddhist reminder to look for whatever was coming around the next bend, to keep an open mind despite the crap of motherhood and genteel college-educated poverty. One of us would carry it for a while. Then, when need arose, one of us would dig it out from our purse or pocket and transfer it to the other like a talisman.

But I didn't want the Open or its message in that moment, couldn't consider exposing my heart to the universe when I already felt shredded and vulnerable.

I picked up the baby from the sitter, swaddled him in layers of polar fleece and knit, wrestled him into the car seat, and drove home. I fed him and put him down for a nap. Then I went to the Internet to search for "serenity no health insurance." I wanted to see the argument and to pick it apart with my brain and my teeth, either to ravage it or to throw myself onto it for safety.

"Your search returned 0 results." Google helpfully offered to amend my query: "Did you mean to search for *Serenity Now Health Insurance?*"

Sure. Even better. Whatever. I clicked on the link. The screen listed Christian Web sites offering group prayer for the ill and private financial assistance for the saved. Several other search terms—a visit to Amazon, a troll through a news database—all turned up nothing. This secret was so underground it was nowhere on the Web.

Fine. I would attend the workshop.

I went back to the co-op a few days later to copy down the date and time, but the poster was gone. No serenity for me.

Health itself was no bedrock, and the body would break in time. But benefits were safety and future—lullaby and go to sleep, my feminist version of Prince Charming on a white horse, love incarnate, the thing that would make me real, would catch me when I fell and set me back on my feet. I could not even think of my life or myself without thinking about my insurance status, and I had narrowed my sense of foundation and tomorrow to the size of a white plastic card that would have fit in my wallet.

How did I get there, and how did we?

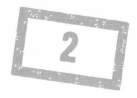

MEDICAL MAGIC

A grade school stomachache meant that Mom picked me up from school and took me home to the midday silence of my room, fully lit with the secret cheer of the weekend in the middle of the week. Childhood sickness itself was a refuge of rest and slowed time. The lazy days of grade school fever or sore throat were sound tracked with the seesaw refrain of *Green Acres*. The television show lulled me into a happy drowse as it pantomimed class conflict as a cultural clash to be smoothed over with the flirtatious purr of attraction to one's opposite.

The show's country setting and characters made no impression on my memories because they seemed ordinary. Didn't everyone want a pet pig? But the character of rich Lisa Douglas fascinated me. Eva Gabor sang in accented staccato, "I just *ah-*DORE a penthouse view. . . . Dah-ling, I love you, but give me Park Avenue!" I figured Park Avenue was somewhere in California. *Penthouse* was a nudie magazine, so what view was she looking for? Gabor's accent made me think she was saying "panchouse," which was, I imagined, something French, maybe a food, or a food you could also live in, like a pumpkin shell *. . . and there he kept her very well.*

Through these slow afternoons, I reveled in the body's ability to concoct its own cures with the ingredients of time, orange juice, and sleep. I conked out between episodes of *The Hulk* (lesson: science and anger will fuck you up) and afternoon reruns of *The People's Court* (lesson: the one with the bad hair was always guilty) and slept through dinnertime, emerging the next morning from hazy dreams with my temperature restored to 98.6 degrees. American sick was vacation, serenaded by the television laugh track.

During those few times when fever or infection got too serious to focus on the television screen, I had to close my eyes and watch the scarier version of sickness in my body's genetic memory. The splotches of color inside my eyelids formed into my roots of sickness, like staring into the vacant eyes of a skull. Fever had once been a killer, stalking the pioneers and mowing down friends and cousins in *Little House on the Prairie*. Pneumonia and infections killed child-aunts and child-uncles in wartime Germany, a family tree filled with Xs. Healthcare is luck, and we are barely alive. Mold made penicillin; because of mold, I got antibiotics for an ear infection and got to live. Even as a child, I stared back over my shoulder down into the void of what if, marveling that I was breathing at all. And the next easy step is a terrible vigilance about healthcare and the body, an appreciation and a grief. I had accidentally cheated by being born late.

In first grade I knocked my arm on the curb in a bike collision and made a greenstick fracture. We drove to Silver Cross Hospital with my arm on a yellow couch cushion. Dr. Duffy set it in warm plaster and wrapped it with a beige Ace bandage. Afterward, Mom took me to Bruns Sales and let me buy a treat. I chose a blue satin flamenco outfit for my Barbie. It had multicolored ruffles down the body and matching blue shoes. Later that night, I remember crying and talking to my mom, saying, "I'm sorry," over and over; and now I wonder what I was apologizing for. Maybe for breaking my body by accident, this body that is not mine, this body that barely got here in one piece.

We had coverage when I was a kid, and Mom says it was easier then and healthcare wasn't as expensive or complicated. We went to the doctor for broken bones and chicken pox. Doctors are busy in their white coats, and the doctor's office is kind of like a hardware store for your body. You show them bumps and rashes, and they give you ointment and shots. There are a lot of things that you don't ask doctors about.

You don't ask about the things in your head. Lying in bed at night, a vivid feeling that would come and go: the molecules of my body expanded until each was a huge electric cloud with me lost in the middle. When it started to happen, I had to wait it out like an alien visitation. Decades later, therapists would tell me it is panic and disassociation, but I had no name for it.

My anxiety did not get its start with health insurance. I am made from anxiety itself. Before there was me, there were threads of doubt and worry about money, work, and healing. Today, when I get a hospital bill, the gap between what I have and what I owe plays a dissonant chord against the song of money sung by my ancestors and handed down to me.

As an accidental and unappointed story carrier, I absorb passed-down moments and I puzzle over them, and they rumble and rumble and rumble around, thump-thump, unbalanced, like tennis shoes in a dryer.

Here is one I can't let go of: My grandmother Sophie, my dad's mom, had to work in a mine in the green hills of southern Germany. She had a long rope of black hair she wound on her head like a basket, and a formal Black Forest outfit with a hat that had massive red pom-poms on it, from another time, back when "folk" meant people. She was young and in love with the postmaster. She needed money to care for her parents. Her mother was a diabetic who needed to get a leg amputated, and her father had been injured in the war and couldn't work.

In the end, Sophie broke off the engagement with her postman because of money, because of healthcare. She married George—who would become my grandfather, Papa—instead of the postmaster, because George promised her money to care for her parents. Then George moved Sophie across the ocean to the green hills of western Arkansas. She kept that postmaster in her heart, echoing the longing in that song my mother sung to me as a child:

> My bonnie lies over the ocean
> Oh bring back my bonnie to me

She baked cakes for extra money in the shape of clowns, footballs, race cars, and guitars. She wrote songs, entered contests, and filled a bookshelf with mail-order Reader's Digest books like *Mysteries of the Unexplained*. She carried a pocket-sized notebook of Spanish vocabulary words that I found in her things after her death, roiled up in a box of Catholic saint metals and rosaries and spindly pairs of metal eyeglass frames. She was learning Spanish, bits at a time.

In the years I scavenged for healthcare, her story came up again to the surface, bobbing with different knots and eyes facing the sun like a rolling, floating log. For want of a nail, the kingdom was lost. For want of healthcare, her life story changed. Love stories—especially the tragic ones—are always about choices. We are supposed to pick our battles, learn from our mistakes. I didn't know how or what to learn from hers.

My brother and my sister and I were all accidents of medical intervention, walking around on borrowed time with broken pieces fixed. My brother was born with pyloric stenosis, a muscle blockage in his stomach, and would have died without surgery. My sister needed penicillin for ear infections. I came out with a hemangioma on my shoulder, a strawberry birthmark they had to cut out. Mom said it would have bled and bled.

The scars that snaked across our pink bodies were raised fingers of caution and strokes of dumb luck. Immunization shots, like time capsules injected beneath the skin, carried the names of diseases past. Polio was a jumble of swimming pools and the iron lung and a wheelchaired president Franklin Delano Roosevelt, all shrunk down to microscopic scale and put into the body like a magic spell. If we lived in the era of medical magic, then it seemed any remaining illnesses were our own fault, self-created as the result of modern weakness. Diagnoses like "nerves" remained the head's catchall for syndromes in which the body reacted to poisons that medicine could not see.

My brother Glenn was in first grade when he went into the hospital for stabbing stomach pains. We went to visit him, and I remember him sitting in the hospital bed coloring neatly with markers in a coloring book laid on a metal table that extended across the high bed.

A doctor came into the room and greeted my parents, then said something like, "Hello, son," to me because I had a short haircut.

"I'm a girl," I said spitefully to the doctor. My brother was getting all the attention and even had a little television on a pneumatic arm next to his bed.

The doctor left. Sometime after that, Glenn hunched over his coloring book, squinting, face all bunched up. The marker slipped into wide arcs as he scrawled furiously across the rough newsprint paper. He ruined the picture, which shocked me. Mom must have rushed to the bed. He was released a few days later with an unclear diagnosis of "nervous stomach."

In the last thirty years, medicine has swung away from blame and toward biology. Both colic and nervous stomach are now seen to be partially caused by defects of biology rather than a person's nervous character. It's important, says the MedHelp Web site, to avoid attributing a series of physical symptoms to anxiety, because that effectively ends the quest for treatment. My brother has accepted his bad stomach as a lifelong condition.

The doctor's mistake in the hospital room tells me that I was
eight, the year of my first short haircut, making that the summer
of 1979, six months before the wild Reagan years in America. Pop
culture records those years as "bright lights, big city," as in the
title of Jay McInerney's novel—big profits of a stock market boom
but also recession. Mom calls the 1980s "the bad decade," a period
of relative money stress and worry for my parents, who owned a
small business. I think of those times and I think about Mom chain-
smoking late at work. The office built on to our house seemed to
have its own stratified atmosphere, filled with a layer of smoke
like the gray of a midwestern winter sky, like the gray circles under
Dad's eyes.

This is not to say I was unhappy. We lived three blocks away from
Cherry Hill School, which had six classrooms—two each for the first,
second, and third grades. I gobbled books and ripped through math
worksheets as fast as I wanted, and there was no one to tell me to
slow down. There was no heaven like reading *Robinson Crusoe* and
making a shoebox diorama, walking to school and carrying it carefully against my chest like a treasure to Baby Jesus. There is no power
greater than that of a third-grade smart girl who knows she's smart,
who's mouthy and bucktoothed, squinty and quick with her brain
and quick with a laugh, hands on hips, before she knows she's date
meat and wife meat, job meat and death meat.

That smart and scrappy girl has marks of trouble to come, like
the hacking cough. When I forgot to bring cough drops, a teacher at
Cherry Hill dug in her desk for an old candy cane for me to suck on.
Maybe it's the allergies I won't discover for decades or my parents'
smoking. Maybe the cough comes from the bad lungs on Mom's
side of the family, where everybody from that coal-mining town has
the *Husten*, the cough.

Third grade to ninth grade meant the slow morphing of a child
into the person I am today, someone who worries. Depending on

your inclination toward blame, you might see this either as a regrettable hobby or as a response to environmental stresses and toxins. I worried that Dad went to work with dangerous radiation stuff. I stared at the radiation-burn illustrations in the safety pamphlets at his office, and I remember the furious, scary scrubbing in the movie *Silkwood* after Cher's character was exposed to radiation. And then she was killed for telling the truth about the danger. In junior high my friends and I each bought one Ocean Pacific T-shirt with a surfer on it and wore them like uniforms, as if to emphasize our own geographical inability to be cool. The shirts said "Hang Loose," and we wore them as we watched the television miniseries *The Day After* to imagine nuclear annihilation.

When I was a freshman in high school, the family doctor asked me to keep a headache journal, and the pattern—focused around one eye, banded around the forehead like a vice, base of the neck—seems now to indicate tension headaches. Neither that doctor nor any specialist afterward asked me if I knew how to manage stress.

I imagine myself in high school, sitting in my Chevy Cavalier with the Targus-brand tape player I paid to have installed that would shoot its eject key into the back seat when you pressed rewind. The girl with her blazer-style '80s gray and white winter coat, Carmex in the pocket, must have seen a diagnosis of "tension" as an accomplishment, I think, and also as an embarrassing by-product of work. Of course I was tense, I may have thought then. I was laser focused on honor roll, college scholarships, schoolbooks, writing, not getting pregnant, not messing up. I was going to pull the slingshot all the way back and launch myself up out of the industrial corn grid into a blank space of somewhere, anywhere, else.

A nurse stuck electrodes all over my scalp with sticky goo, and the scribbled tracks on a graph paper roll showed some sort of micro-seizures. Electrodes stuck to my chest showed a heart murmur, so the doctor put me on a drug called a beta-blocker. I don't know if it helped. It seemed to, but so did Advil. The doctor ordered an MRI, a new and expensive procedure in the mid-1980s, to look for a tumor. The metal rack slid back into the round opening with me strapped in. I watched the beige-coated metal of the tube as it began to spin around me and ricocheted with a deafening, hammering sound.

I got to keep the films of the meat x-ray of my tumorless head, which looked like a bisected cabbage, layers of me all the way to the center with nowhere to hide. And I knew it was me immediately, something so intimate about the inside of the mouth, the cathedral ceiling's ridged imprint from my pink plastic dental retainer. That's my nose, there, with the bump, and the slope of the forehead, and the lips pulled tight around the buckteeth wrapped in braces. What that bisected cabbage doesn't show is a layer of money. As I look back into my body's formation, I see the thread of that damning abstraction, currency, like buckshot riffling the skin. We are altered shapes, like trees whose trunks and branches have grown in and through a chain-link fence. I am a strange meat sculpture with twists and knots and curlicues toward the top.

The word *worry* has roots in the Old High German verb *wurgen*, "to strangle." The body seizes up and knots after too much exposure to worry or tension. What I don't know is whether worry causes these ailments or whether certain bodies are born with seeds of trouble, sites where worry can latch on and take hold. The past and the present come together in the body, and the body tries to make sense of them and knit them together. Like an amateur car mechanic, I make guesses about my family's bodies. Maybe my brother's nervous stomach is linked to the pyloric stenosis in his infancy. Maybe my shoulder and jaw pain, even my headaches, are connected by levers and pulleys to the scar along my right shoulder. I like these physical explanations better than the alternative theory that somehow our anxious minds have invisibly made our bodies sick because emotion caused muscles to flood with stress hormones and the ensuing chain reaction of repeated episodes led to permanent reshaping and, some might say, damage. Because we don't see or understand the levers and pulleys of the mind, we assume that the space in our skulls is empty, pliable, and shapeable. An anxiety-related condition seems to leak from the brain out into my body, and I am an inadequate sculptor of myself. Alternatively, you might see my body as a fossilized piece of corporate healthcare, the body shaping the brain that forms the words to tell this tale.

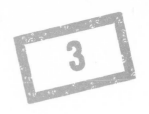

DO IT YOURSELF

The paramedics lifted me onto a stretcher and shouted to my friends, "Has she used any illegal drugs?"

I had passed out after my first panic attack, summer of 1991 after my second year of college. The ER nurses in Northfield, Minnesota, who cut open my T-shirt didn't know what was wrong, and neither did I. The doctors stuck electrodes to my scalp but couldn't find anything wrong with my physical brain.

I checked out of the hospital after a few days, thinking I was cured. My friend Liz came to drive me home, and we laughed as I carried my bag of clothes toward the glass double doors of the hospital lobby. I remember looking back at the billing and reception woman in that teal-carpeted lobby with the particleboard partitions and desks. I stopped to give her my parents' insurance card. I had the strange sense of playing child, of the end of dependence. This was a last fling in which my body could do what it wanted and someone else would pick up the tab. I knew, too, that there would be a bill, and I had the vague but solid guilt that my parents would be asked to pay for a mistake in my head that I couldn't solve with willpower.

Panic attacks multiplied that summer by exponentials I could not track, a string of them like staggered reflections in two facing mirrors. I went home to the attic apartment I shared with Liz and two other college friends, where we baked our own bread to save money and ate generic Cheerios with apple juice. We believed in the curative powers of simplicity and attention. When I felt my lungs fold inward, I moaned in frustration and one of these lovely, steadfast friends would drop whatever she was doing, set down her book or stop mixing dinner, and run to be with me. They watched my breathing, held my hand, worried as I did about the possible causes of this inability to breathe. Living with panic means living in a cloud of anxiety. Because of the stress of that summer, those friendships were never the same. I caused too much worry I couldn't pay back. I liked being the strong girl in that group, and we knew each other by our muscles and boldness. But in a panic attack on that floor I was weak.

We watched the world and its chemicals with anxiety; we believed that part of our job was to turn away from what was made in a lab, to help point the world toward a freedom it had forgotten. I drove up to work each day as an intern at the Minnesota Department of Agriculture, where I interviewed farmers who were trying to go organic about their changing views on putting chemicals in the soil. Liz was in the early stages of getting sick with ulcerative colitis, a disorder that would plague her for a decade; she and I had met as co-organizers of the environmental group on campus. We worked together on a support committee for a local factory that made computer components, and some of the workers developed lung infections and neurological disorders. A physics professor on campus had graphed the local cancer cluster that was invisible on the picturesque postcards sold in the campus bookstore.

It wasn't safe to drive because I kept blacking out. I quit the internship, and Mom drove up from Chicago to take me to the Mayo Clinic in southeast Minnesota.

We waited to be seen by a resident, who looked me over, listened to my chest, and said, "It's probably in your head." He was in a rush; I don't hold it against him now.

He was right, but that didn't help at the time.

I went out to the car with my mom and sat in the back seat, staring at the silver knob of the door lock. I imagined two solutions: I would buy myself a gun and kill myself. Or I would move out to Wyoming, get a waitressing job, and start a new life. Both extremes were motivated by the shame of having my body paralyzed by my head.

Back home in New Lenox, Illinois, I waited for an appointment with the Chicago neurologist and paged through my copy of *Our Bodies, Ourselves*, a phone book–sized reference on women's health replete with blurry '70s photos of women who touched their pregnant bellies, stretched their aging bodies, or took their blood pressure while wearing turtlenecks. I lay on my bed and paged aimlessly, scanning symptoms of every disorder. Could a fetus be causing this wooziness? Or a brain tumor? Mono? AIDS?

I met my best friend from high school, Nicki, before she went away for sophomore year of school. We ate fried spinach pie with ketchup at a Greek place called Mickey's, and we licked the grease from our fingers.

"Maybe I'm pregnant," I said.

"But you took a test," she said.

Pregnant would be an easy fix, because then at least something positive would come from this. On the other hand, if I was dying, that meant there would be nothing else to worry about.

What I loved about my friends was that they seemed to all develop a picture of me in which my secrets were revealed. "You worry too much," Nicki probably said, leveling her dark eyes at me as she sat wrapped in flannel in that greasy restaurant. She would smile at me because she knew she was right. Once, she had given me two mice for a birthday because, as she said, "You need some mice." And every time she said it—"You worry too much"—it was a new revelation, an insight I had marveled over and forgotten about again. Yes, that is right. You know me as I do not know myself.

The neurologist found nothing wrong with my brain. In the clear gray truth of that August, I went back up to Minnesota to find as near to Wyoming or suicide as a good girl could stomach. The counselor diagnosed panic, a disorder that doesn't really describe causes or outcomes. I had worries and tendencies and various predispositions, and I could make lists of scenarios and of the contents of my charts. Like one in three women, I had been assaulted by a guy who defined what he was doing as sex. Details and experiences cohere into stories and theories, but the details are akin to individual cuts and stray bacteria. For my purposes, they mislead. I want to forsake those trees for this particular forest, to stay with that young woman's body, with the permanent marks and the healthcare needs those marks created.

The counselor wanted to give me a chemical cure, a little blue pill she said would make it all go away. I refused and found myself in the rush of the first week of classes, crouched against the wall in a hallway of the student union with another panic attack. Another at dinner, another the next morning, and getting across campus became a logistical challenge. In that tunnel vision the choices narrowed and simplified: school or no school? School wouldn't work, not like this.

I shouldered into that problem, felt the burn in my life and my muscles as I ripped myself from one track to another, knowing I would end up winded but somewhere else. I found a room to rent in Minneapolis and asked Mom for a loan. She said no, which I respected then and still respect today. Mom had the right to tell me to stay in school, and I had the right to leave as long as I footed the bill for my own adventure. She went through bouts of pure hatred for her job as office manager for my dad's health physics company. Mom had a Post-it note on her desk that was faded by the sun. It had the number eight on it, then crossed out, then the number seven, crossed out, then six, counting down the years she had left to work until all of her kids were done with college. Fifteen years after my college graduation, she's still there, working for health insurance.

While Mom tracked her employment in years of dread in South Side Chicago, I got a coffee shop job that blustery fall of 1991 in Minneapolis and celebrated the Mayday liberated space of community bookstores and radical art collectives and birthday cakes for dead anarchists. The small bookshelf in my rented room also held volume 4 of the *Foxfire* series, an illustrated guide to rural folk knowledge containing instructions on how to tan leather, how to build a wood fence and a homemade banjo. I would never consider devoting an afternoon to tanning a hide, yet I liked knowing it was an option. I also owned an illustrated paperback field guide entitled *Edible Wild Plants*, although I never used it to forage for anything I actually ate. Knowing I could eat dandelion greens or rose hips was enough for me.

The 1970s response to money stress was to make your own cost-free solutions: plant a garden, sew your clothes. I was an artsy-craftsy do-it-yourselfer, raised in that decade by a thrifty mom to weave macramé plant hangers by following the instructions in a library book. So my immersion in anarchist culture of the upper Midwest in the early 1990s felt like a homecoming. Self-published punk zines, independent performance projects, squats, and urban gardens all felt as familiar, somehow, as woven potholders and homemade pickles.

I carefully unpacked my stack of political tracts, health-related reference tomes, and women's health zines with hand-drawn pages explaining how to make an herbal tea to cure a urinary tract infection or to induce an abortion. It was the early 1990s, and the Internet was still the domain of people wearing cloaks and quoting *The Hitch-hiker's Guide to the Galaxy*. Paper still carried the critical weight of precious information.

I worked behind the counter at the coffee shop with a dancer named Arwen. She rode her bike in the rain and drank soymilk from a mustard container she reclaimed from the trash. When she sniffled with a cold, she ate garlic cloves. When I rubbed my aching sinuses, she fed me massive green tablets.

"It's spirulina," she said, blue eyes twinkling like the elf she is. "It's green algae. It's *super* good for you."

Arwen needed massages for her dancer's muscles, and when I picked her up in the Cavalier sleepy-eyed from one of those appointments, she said, "You should try it. It's so lovely."

I recoiled in horror at the thought of a stranger's hands on my bare skin. Nature-loving hippie boys at college had offered back rubs as a shortcut to friendly making out. When they grabbed for my right shoulder—the site of my hemangioma scar, a rippled chunk of muscle that never relaxes—I flinched and turned myself sideways beyond their hands.

"Jesus, you're tense," they might have said with sympathy, confusion, or the slightest hint of blame. "Relax. Chill out, man."

I relaxed in the mosh pit at crashing punk shows with elbows flying. I went to First Ave with my friend Steve, the musician who was also taking an extended break from school and sleeping in a basement next to an ancient furnace that looked like an octopus. Steve hosted an "orphan Thanksgiving" for everybody who wasn't going home. In that house full of boys, we ate falafel and random casseroles in a hand-over-hand crowd in his threadbare living room. He and his friends had bought a box of plastic Jabba the Hutt heads from a local surplus store, and a chorus line of Jabbas dotted the window sills and mantel. Thank God for punk rock, which made it sort of wistful and Westerbergian when Steve had a seizure and fell on his nose in his kitchen, blood everywhere and no insurance, or when he got a bookstore job so he could go on a binge of dental work before he quit.

I began to entrust my health to the patchwork safety net of community health practitioners, the workers at Planned Parenthood and various other free clinics, the herbologists and hobby homeopaths working at the community co-ops. I also turned to the volunteer-led women's center support groups and to the crisis hotlines. I knew—or thought I knew—that if I did not choose a life path that would end in an office cubicle, I would be responsible for my own body. I would have to learn how to take care of it along with the sometimes-correct guesses from friends and strangers. And that has pretty much proven correct, though I think this burden is something no person should have to handle. The ideal of self-sufficiency was comforting as I leapt away from my parents' healthcare plan and prepared for survival in a wild and foreign frontier. The DIY ethic combined with my class-warfare perspective to create a virulent hatred of healthcare institutions in which I equated doctors with debt and the Man, as if a hospital were a heavily guarded glass vault set up to taunt me with the jewel of healthcare.

The biting cold of Minnesota in January 1992 brought my vision into tight focus. I could see again. Because I knew I could leave again if I needed to, I went back to school. That spring, I met my anarchist friends J—— and Mike at a deli in our college town. A few minutes later, a union steward and another two workers from the local computer-components factory came in, and we shook hands all around. Within an hour, we had made notes for a community forum and sketched out the lineup of speakers. We recruited a professor from campus and a community member to talk about the growing range of safety concerns with the plant.

The day of the panel, I walked up a hill fifteen minutes before the event. J—— and Mike had been there early setting up. I could see the local elementary school, which had its doors propped open. The sun was out and the bushes were budding with green. I stopped at a driveway halfway to the school and felt my throat constrict. I felt a million miles away, as if my head had been mailed to another place.

I was with J—— or my boyfriend or someone else in our group, and I must have told that person at the last minute that I couldn't go in. It was a room full of people, and I didn't want to ruin the event by crying in the middle of it. What I wanted was to be inside that gym with the shiny floor and the red and blue tape lines on the linoleum, and wanting it and being angry at my own head only made the panic worse.

"I gotta go," I said to whoever was with me. "Let me know how it turns out." I turned corners and traced green rectangles along the sidewalk grid, the only way I knew to calm down.

That spring, I relented and took the sky blue antidepressants. I felt a chemical buzz as the pills settled into my head and moved the furniture around. My brain had artificial components, in a community where real and authentic were prized above all else; I had to make a practical choice. My chemical-free brain shut down my body, and I missed classes, parties, jobs, and large swathes of time. Artificial seemed better than dead or useless.

In the summer of 1992, between my junior and senior year, I enrolled in an anarchist institute in the green hills of Vermont, hoping to burrow into the anarchist universe and hollow out a permanent home. But my East Coast smiley, gangly college boyfriend helped me develop a urinary tract infection before he left for Italy, and I spent most of the summer collecting recipes for medicinal teas and juices in my women's health guides. Peeing fire, I conducted a women's health-clinic tour of the East Coast. In rural Vermont I resorted to repeated and expensive emergency room visits, begging rides from strangers and fellow students at the school where I was supposed to be studying. The harried nurses and doctors, busy with tractor injuries and power-tool wounds, lost my results and my records, then apologized for giving me the wrong antibiotics after red splotchy hives crept up my arms and down my legs. I slept on any couch I could find and read women's health pamphlets about the urinary tract.

To comfort myself and to create an illusion of control, I bought *Where There Is No Doctor*, a public health guide created for people living in rural Latin America. The book featured line drawings of shortish, brown-skinned peasants in wide-brimmed hats, the women with black hair in braids, calmly treating naked *compañeros* with nasty-looking lumps and animal bites. Desperate, I made a retreat to the midwestern comforts of home. And the infection eventually went away by itself.

After college was done in 1993, I headed east with that gangly, smiley New York boyfriend. We chose Boston because it was not as big as New York and because his parents had fallen in love there. One might wonder: upon graduation from college with no plan and a confirmed anxiety disorder, why move far away to a strange city where traffic looped in mad whirlpools of death? I want to summon my former self for a chat about this issue, but she is so driven to force away these problems with willpower and effort through a concerted and self-designed immersion therapy program that she won't listen to me at all as I pretend to be so much wiser now. I found a job for $6.50 an hour at a photo processing and graphic design shop, and my boyfriend found a horrible job for $5.00 an hour at an Italian restaurant.

If you were alive in a time before Google, you remember going to a new city and stopping at a sidewalk hamburger place on a street where you were lost or where the houses looked kind of cool. You might lean over the counter and ask the busy cook at the grill, "Excuse me, can you tell me where the post office is?" You sketch a map as you listen, then use the pay phone to make calls from the real estate section of the classifieds in the Sunday paper. At the coffee shop down the street, you ask for directions to the library. If there's a library, all will be well. You camp out at a roomy, sunlit square table in the corner with a priceless treasure: the phone book. You page through it slowly, taking notes in a spiral notebook, a few words and a few numbers, anything that might serve to create a life. You make calls from the pay phone at the corner Laundromat to get the phone turned on.

I think I found the Boston Women's Center either in the phone book under "W" or on a flyer at the food co-op. I called and got directions from a frazzled, volunteer part-time receptionist. I took the T to Central Square in Cambridge and followed my map to a rambling Victorian house with peeling lilac paint supporting a row of scraggly sunflowers. I walked in, shoulders curled inward, afraid to bump into anything that might jar this illusion of support and make it disappear. A side kitchen offered a shelf crammed with cardboard boxes of tea in different flavors. A row of clipboards overstuffed with flyers advertised places to rent, notices for events, and workshops. I found a rape survivors' support group. It was free. I attended for a few months, skirting the edges of that place, making a few friends. I was so hesitant to even believe free help existed—that they wanted nothing from me in return.

Without insurance, I'd taken myself off antidepressants, so panic and depression had returned with a rumbling momentum. I could see their shapes in my peripheral vision on the bus. During rush hour on the T, going home, bodies bumped against mine. With the whiff of cheap beer on someone's warm breath from behind me, I was gone. The lights went from yellow to blue, and in my head I was freaking myself out even worse than I needed to, *Goddamn it, I hate this, fuck, keep breathing, keep calm for fuck's sake and no one will notice, I fucking hate this, just fucking breathe.*

When I started to cry on my way home from work, attracting the attention of my fellow riders who offered seats and shoulder pats, I knew I needed to do something. My boyfriend was away working at his new coffee shop job, and I'd been freaking out so badly in the past few days that I'd been sleeping in the bathtub for reasons I can't explain. What I did not realize was that I was dealing with two crises at once: an insurance gap and a mental health emergency. And these are probably not the best foundation for a romantic postcollege relationship in a new city.

Depression was home ground, something I could manage with daily bribes of coffee and the distraction of reading and with pills if it got bad. But panic made a scene. It numbed my hands, put invisible fingers around my throat, tightened my chest muscles, shallowed my breathing, and depleted the oxygen content of my blood until I could not think clearly. Panic attacks created a sense of physical weakness, a wariness, that led to a tentative approach, which seemed to bring on the next panic attack.

I looked under "R" in the phone book and found Rape Crisis Center, because I didn't know whom else to call and the suicide hotline seemed a bit too desperate.

I listened to the recorded message and spoke into the recorder: "My name is Sonya. I just need to talk to someone to get some information."

The woman called me back within a half hour, and I sat alone in the apartment with my forehead on the floor as I talked. I was comforted by the dark cave my head and hair made with the wood and by the reverberation of my voice against the shiny hardwood floor—an unending fascination and sign of high-class living for a midwesterner.

"Are you in a safe place?" asked the woman on the other end of the phone.

"Yeah, I'm in a safe place," I said. "But this happened a long time ago."

"Do you want to talk about it?"

I met her nice, soft voice with a serrated edge of raw need. "No." I sobbed. "I mean, I need a lot more than that. I have to build—I have to get people here. I need names."

"Do you have insurance?"

No, I answer. Of course not. She gave me a list of names, therapists who were taking new patients and who offered a sliding scale fee structure.

"Thank you so much for calling me back," I said, crying. "Thank you so much."

She was a bit puzzled. "This is what we do."

"But if you weren't here . . . if you weren't here . . ."

"Don't worry about that. We are. Call back if you need help."

Like a fluffy little yippy dog, panic requires frequent shampooing and grooming by a cadre of professionals. To accessorize and maintain my panic in the manner to which it had become accustomed, I paid the lowest end of full price for therapy, $85 a week; for periodic visits to a psychiatrist; and for medication. No one mentioned charity care or sliding scale programs for the psychiatric visits or for the meds, and I didn't know to ask. I spent almost as much each month on mental health as I did on rent, which left about $350 a month for food, utilities, and everything else.

Boston—the name of the city now makes me shiver, but I'm not sure whether it's with pride at survival or remembered dread at the intensity of everything I learned during my self-imposed domestic study-abroad program. The word *Boston* now connotes a physical experience: moving, walking, through the circulatory system of the T underground, looping and finding directions, reading the newspaper to ferret out events and organizations and resources, walking home late at night from work, walking home from the Dollar Store with my bags of shampoo and aspirin and Ziploc bags, meeting the Food Not Bombs kids who scavenged in the Dumpsters and cooked food to feed the homeless and themselves, perfecting as I did the fine art of urban scavenging. Did it have to be this way? I wondered then—as I still wonder—whether I'd maneuvered myself into this lack, whether the anxiety I felt in these surroundings was of my own creation or something larger.

That fall, I lost a contact lens, so I made an appointment with an eye doctor in a fancy-looking mall in an old, ornate building off Boylston in downtown Boston. After the eye exam, they set me up with my new lenses in their little glass vials and a container of saline solution. I palmed one, rinsed it with a squirt, and dropped it in my eye, blinking as the world swam underwater and then eased into crisp focus.

I smiled at the doctor's assistant, who asked me how they felt.

"Great," I said, taking out my checkbook. I was happy to pay because these were my eyes, I had enough money, and now I could see.

"What health plan do you have?" she asked, turning to her computer.

I told her I didn't have insurance, and she winced as she gave me a total. I wrote the check, and as I tore it out, I heard plastic rustling. I looked up to see that she had loaded a huge bag of virtually every contact lens product she could put her hands on in that store. She doesn't know that fifteen years later I am still running on the fuel of that moment. I still remember the glint of that beige plastic bag with the green letters. I remember the kindness of strangers.

Snow fell that first Boston November of 1993, and my boyfriend burned with fever. I bought him orange juice and smoothed his forehead as I pretended to be Florence Nightingale. My boyfriend's dad was a famous doctor at Memorial Sloan-Kettering in New York City. We called, he listened to the boyfriend's symptoms, diagnosed a case of strep, and called in a prescription to a pharmacy.

My throat pinched with strep and my head swam, but the boyfriend's dad would not call in a prescription for me. Was it because he was a Catholic and I was living in sin with his son, having daily sin with him on our queen-sized mattress, laid right on the hardwood floor of our one-bedroom apartment? More likely, the doctor thought it was too risky or improper to diagnose a nonrelative over the phone. I think the doctor suggested I go to Boston General for the free care program. I can't remember if I got angry. Maybe I was too sick to waste the energy. Maybe, given my worship of healthcare as a wrathful and remote deity, I found it inconceivable to yell at or beg a New York doctor.

I bundled up to ride the T to the "free clinic"—the words had an ominous sound. I'd never encountered free healthcare, and I assumed that if they were giving it away, you'd have to endure some public humiliation first. My midwestern suburban head bubbled with visions of an island leprosy clinic: people in rags shuffling about, moaning as their limbs dropped off behind them, as Newt Gingrich popped up from behind the waiting room seats with a hunter's cap and a shotgun to take aim.

But the hospital was easy to find, and the waiting room was quiet, if a little musty. The maize 1970s decor needed an update, as did the crumpled back issues of *Cat Fancy* magazines. But when I asked for a charity-care application, nobody blasted an air horn and called me a loser. I got a chair and clipboard to myself and a fluorescent-lit drop ceiling over my head. No trapdoor opened to whisk me down a twisty slide to hell to be pricked with used heroin needles by the disembodied evil twin of a judgmental Ronald Reagan. I filled out the empty spaces on the intake sheet, including the space for "income." You can sort of guess you're poor if you don't know your annual salary before multiplying by forty and fifty-two. I located the figure on the chart below, which told me that I qualified for free care.

A nurse touched the back of my throat with a swab and said she'd call with the results. I rode the T home through the snow in that foreign city, watching cars' headlights hollow out yellow cones in the muffling gray spray. The entire city seemed to sizzle with the noise of black wheels peeling against wet pavement. The subway lurched and I curled into the plastic seat.

I quit the photo place after a few months and signed up with a temp agency, which offered me more money and the possibility of benefits. I was assigned to an HMO clinic—no health insurance myself—where I sat at a gray Formica desk and held an angular black phone receiver to my ear. I called orthopedic patients to remind them about their upcoming appointments. "Don't forget your 3:00, you lucky bastard."

I read the fine print on my weekly Manpower time sheet and realized that in order to get the benefits they described, I'd have to work for months in a continuous contract. The moment you dipped under forty hours a week, you lost benefits eligibility. If they didn't call you for work one day, you were ineligible for a month. And the benefits were so expensive anyway that I barely made enough to pay for them, so I didn't bother.

That winter of 1994, I got a real job as an overnight counselor at a group home for teens, and it seemed real life started now: I won health insurance, a policy in my name, my first card. My folder of benefits information contained a pamphlet from the Employee Assistance Program, a 1-800 number I could call to talk with a stranger for fifteen minutes, after which time I would apparently hang up with a renewed commitment to workplace productivity. I never tried that, and I don't remember having mental health benefits—either that or I was so new to insurance that I imagined secret messages would be sent from therapists directly to my bosses: "The new one you hired is a loony."

Maybe I imagined the group home would be a gentle after-school-special moment of me changing the lives of a few teens. Instead, I found the opposite: a gauntlet of swearing and furniture throwing and suicide attempts and messes and blood and police sirens. But something about my shyness—my panic itself—wanted to be thrown in and pureed by the edges of that place. And I knew, too, that panic and depression were real there. I ended up learning a lot about my own symptoms and how to manage them as I sat in employee trainings designed to help us help our cases.

I broke up with my college boyfriend, probably because the stress of our Boston adventure had shredded all affection between us. I could have moved back to the Midwest, but I'd just started this interesting job and I'd finally started making real friends. I moved in with Monica, one of the other counselors at the group home, a badass with long blonde hair and a black leather jacket who said "fuck you" as a cheerful greeting. She would one day be a lawyer and a mother of two, but in that moment, she was my survival role model. I watched her navigate interactions with administrators, staring them down and rolling her eyes. She took me out for breakfast after my night shift ended. After a few of our conversations about our families, she pointed me in the direction of Linda, who she said was the best shrink in Boston for people like us.

I went to a party thrown by someone I knew through the women's center and met Brooke, whose hilarious self-deprecation confounded my stereotypes of confident, smooth-talking easterners. We identified each other within five minutes as fellow neurotic anarchists. What's more, she also worked at a group home and had edited an anarchist magazine in college. She was convinced that if she, a New York Jewish lesbian, ever went to the Midwest, she'd be instantly killed by marauding rednecks. Her fear of *schmutz* and germs, paired with her desire for social revolution, wove us together around coffee shop tables—two worried, agonized, self-doubting firebrands.

At work I spent a good part of midnight to 6 a.m., six days a week, in a place we called the alcove. It was a little nook in a bay window on the second floor of a twisty, Victorian house in Cambridge. Sometimes I talked to the teenagers who woke up with nightmares.

At night I vacuumed and straightened the staff office of the youth home in the 3 a.m. quiet. Leaning with my shoulder, I pushed the vacuum nozzle forward, then pulled backward at a slant, starting at the hips. Push, pull, above the roar that was strangely peaceful, like the ocean. Often when I was vacuuming the thin gray carpeting in the front office, my body would call forth snippets of memory from the various places I'd vacuumed. Not at home, which didn't count, but the bumping of the vacuum head, the coiling of the cord, in various workplaces and apartments: Mom and Dad's office, Pizza Hut, the video store, dorm rooms and hallways, coffee shops, bookstores, the photo store lobby. Always with the feeling that uncoiling the cord of a vacuum cleaner was strangely intimate, a quiet-time ritual bridging the places of home and work. In the kitchen I made myself a gut-burning concoction of triple-strength Nescafé, hot water, and cocoa, then scrubbed the metal teapot, filigreed with brown whirls of burned grease, until it shone.

At around 6 until 8 a.m., I cooked breakfast and laid the foundation for the day's order in the house. In Maslow's hierarchy of needs, a landmark in humanist psychology, a person cannot meet higher needs until the basic biological needs are met. The group home was an ordered environment to provide food and shelter but also a sense of security so the residents could work on attachment and family conflicts. I built the bottom layer of the pyramid, and those silent, unseen tasks of caring for a house reminded me of every family member I had ever loved. My grandparents, my parents, knew and know how to butcher, how to can and preserve, how to cut down a tree, build a house, and find water. During college and after, I comforted myself through the separation from the familiar with work that required deft movements: scraping glops of food from a drain in food service, tying the knot on a garbage bag, flattening a box, stacking books, clearing a table and swiping coins into my apron pocket. I rely on my hands and, in work situations, I know they are reliable.

Brooke and I met in our favorite coffee shop, the Someday Café, to work on an article about our experiences as direct care workers. We criticized the care given to our clients and the overreliance on medication, but we also listed the ways in which the structures of the job were hard on the workers. We listed the injuries, the emotional stress, and the low pay of the mental healthcare system. Around this same time, I was randomly calling huge union locals and asking if they would come organize our facility, but our staff size was too small for most organizers to bother with.

I contented myself with venting my spleen in writing and with hanging in my office cubby the Wobblies' Cat—a symbol of the old-fashioned International Workers of the World, a semi-anarcho-syndicalist movement from the turn of the last century with a black cat hissing, hackles raised, and the logo, "An Injury to One Is an Injury to All."

We visited another anarchist friend at his new job—a wonkish office downtown where they were organizing for single-payer healthcare. I wanted to run away from the office within five minutes of stepping in the door and standing near the copier. I felt a panic coming on the moment I started to think about the huge task of knocking on doors, telling people how much our healthcare system sucked. The idea of changing that system seemed so laughably massive, especially if the method involved a clipboard instead of a firebomb. I had no

idea, of course, that the slow work of the clipboard and the work
of Mass-Care, launched in 1995, would still be around fifteen years
later, nudging for adequate universal healthcare in that state.

I paged the answering service to get in touch with Linda, my therapist,
and the eaves above me slanted downward, forming a nook where
I liked to hide in the break room on the locked third floor at work. I
had been promoted from overnight staff to regular counselor and
had a caseload, a pay raise, and a buffet of constant conflict to fill
all the hours of the day. The plastic phone—the kind available only
to mental health nonprofits in the mid-nineties and only available in
bulk and in beige—felt cheap and thin, as if it would take an act of
massive faith to accept that healing words could pull me together,
make me work tonight.

I gripped the set of heavy keys hanging from the lanyard around
my neck and listened to the thumps and muffled screams and shouts
from downstairs. Chore time meant slamming doors and yelling,
the outline of staff commands like, "Give me that Lemon Pledge;
there will be no huffing of furniture polish in the back parking lot."
Several of my cases had panic and anxiety disorders, and several of
them were panicking the shit out of me.

The phone rang, and Linda's West Virginia accent settled my nerves
more effectively than a Klonopin omelet. She asked me how I was and
reminded me of all the strategies I knew to deal with the breathing
problem. I could hear the smile in her voice. "Awww, honey," she
said, wistful and wise, as if she knew a mental health technique did
not address the weirdness, the humor, and the sadness of the brain.
I heard her exhale cigarette smoke. "You gonna be okay tonight?"

"Yeah," I said. We both laughed because we knew I was both lying
and telling the truth.

Linda said "Awww, honey" a lot that fall. "Stay here, stay in your
body," she said when I called her in a panic.

Monica's two-year contract at the group home ended, and few of us could handle the place for longer than that. She moved on to a job at Starbucks—with benefits—while she researched law school applications. Every night when she closed, she brought home plastic garbage bags filled with pastries that had been destined for the Dumpster. Since she was moving up in the world, she passed on Linda's "cleaning scholarship" to me.

In return for a fee discount on group therapy, I arrived weekly to clean during the daytime, when the gray wash of weak Boston sun revealed the therapy room with its guard down. I opened the blinds and moved about the room with no pressure to verbalize or make sense. I wiped the city soot from the window sills and believed I was performing a rite both sacred and prosaic, like a monk in a monastery scrubbing a pot.

I dumped a mound of my therapist's lipstick-smudged cigarette butts into the trash, then spritzed Windex into the ashtray and wiped it clean. The ashtray lived on the window sill in a little parallelogram-shaped closet alcove that jutted from the main therapy room of Linda's office. In the evenings, when she was between clients, Linda often stood in the alcove and tapped a Benson & Hedges from its pearly box. She flicked the lighter as she held the cigarette tight between puckered, coral-lipsticked lips in a way that made her look like a five-foot, very well-dressed pirate. She blew smoke out over the fire escape.

Sometimes, cleaning at Linda's, I watched my own arm, clad in flannel, wiping Windex from a glass tabletop. I looked at the wad-ded paper towel—always in surprise—to see how much dirt could hide on a clear surface. What was strange was the fact that I was cleaning in Boston, on Newbury Street, a fancy shopping district lined with buildings all brick and colonial and twisty, with spires and crazy cupolas and onion-topped steeples, with tectonic-like rises and falls in the woodwork and the floors, with shiny layers of paint on the trim and the banisters, with hallways that curled and rose and fell and met at seventy-four-degree angles.

Cleaning means being trusted with a set of keys or a security code. Cleaning means being part of the invisible crowd that mothers a building in the off-hours. Cleaning means building a city in the sense that if we did not dig it back out layer by layer each night, each week, it would become swallowed in minute increments by the earth.

Cleaning in Germany, in Illinois, in Arkansas made sense to my body; these were the places on earth that gathered the molecules I was made from. Cleaning in Boston meant shuffling molecules of soil that felt and smelled foreign. As they buffeted me and swirled as I dusted, I bathed in strangeness. This always reminded me: I chose this. I chose a city at random, seemingly for the purpose of using myself as a science experiment to test whether a life could be built from nothing.

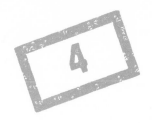

FAILURE TO HEAL

At age twenty-five, I woke one morning in 1996 in Dorchester, a neighborhood in south Boston, with a hollow ache shooting from mouth to nasal cavity. The pain ricocheted inside my skull. I wrapped my fingers around my face and pressed into my flesh. I was still working at the group home, so I had health insurance but no dental. One roommate suggested whiskey. I rubbed some Anbesol on my gums. Friends offered lint-covered and thrice-gifted pain pills from old roommates' sprained ankles and rotator cuff surgeries. My newest boyfriend, whom I'll call Dennis the Red Menace, knew his way around the free healthcare programs offered by the state of Massachusetts. He took me down the street to the community health clinic next to the Dorchester Boys and Girls Club.

I had met Dennis in a meeting organized to plan a counterdemonstration to an upcoming Klan march. I was there to write an article, and Dennis came as a representative of a socialist group. He gave me a ride home and asked for my number, and I thought it was hilarious that this guy—thirteen years older than me, with a kid—would hit on me. His persistence and his bookshelf of labor history won me over. He took me to my first labor picket, and he organized strike support for area workers as effortlessly as other people did their laundry. He taught me about socialism, which I had feared for years but turned to

in secret fascination because the anarchists in my network seemed
surprisingly chaotic. Socialist revolution struck me as a big and sexy
do-it-ourselves project; let's make new countries. Dennis assigned
me readings and bought me beer, and I moved in with him, to the
chagrin of Brooke and my other anarchist friends.

The receptionist at the health clinic handed me a charity-care application. I filled in the spaces and boxes.

Education: BA in Sociology/Anthropology

Income: $16,500.

Position and place of employment: Counselor at a residential
teen center.

Hours per week: Full time.

The receptionist glanced at the income line, took out her stamp,
and smacked it on the top of the form. "Okay," she said. "Here's your
temporary card. Your permanent card will arrive in the mail in three
to six weeks." She didn't make me beg for special dispensation, call
my parents, or shake her head and sigh.

I went upstairs to sit in the waiting room on the health clinic's second floor. The walls of the public health posters about immunizations were printed in Spanish, English, Russian, and Vietnamese.
The mysterious rounded curls of Vietnamese characters reminded
me of the time in childhood before I could read but ached to, of the
distance between meaning and printed language, when letters were
only weighty lines and circles. And I was a child here, twenty-five
but needy, failing, generously yet anonymously taken in to be cared
for by strangers.

I was not exactly ashamed for joining the ranks of "the poor,"
whom I desperately respected in an abstract sense for their grit and
fortitude. Varied in their occupations and ways of scraping by, people
without much cash were legion in my acquaintance. But the poor
remained in my mind a clip-art seventies graphic of a proud-looking

black woman with a pregnant belly and a stylish batik headband wrapped around a natural do. I was not that woman, so I was embarrassed only on my own behalf. As I saw it, I had been given quite a launch toward social success, and yet I managed to stumble to this place on the sputtering firepower of my own ineptitude.

The dental hygienist called me into an examination room and motioned me toward the tilted chair. She strung the clip-on bib behind my neck and left me to study the rustic interior design scheme. To the left of the chair hung a photo of a dark-haired man perched on a Jet Ski and wearing a swimsuit, lifejacket, and sunglasses, with a profusion of chest hair sprouting from the middle and sides of the lifejacket. On the wall facing me, a large preserved fish curled stiffly from its wooden plaque as if breaking through the surface of an invisible pond. The shelf below the fish held hiking photos, a stuffed bird, and a fern. The wall around the Jet Ski photo was covered with images of fishing, hunting, and camping. I also seem to remember a stuffed deer head with a rack of antlers, but that seems insane.

A judicious dental consumer might have taken these decorations as signals of occupational reluctance and disinterest, like a bumper sticker that read, "I'd rather be . . ." At the time, however, I was relieved I'd found a cool dentist.

I knew he was my dentist the moment he walked in because his smile matched the Jet Ski photo, though his hairy chest was covered with his scrubs and robe. I want to write that he set to my mouth as if building a campfire, but I don't remember anything so specific about his skills. He picked at my teeth as I writhed, but he didn't unleash any dental-guilt sermon about the state of my molars. He wasn't interested in shaming me to alter my future behavior toward my teeth. He treated them as a geological problem.

After the x-rays, he clipped the film to a lighted board and hmmmed, tapping his pen and writing codes on my chart. He then sat down on his padded twirly stool, clasped his hands across his lap, and described the terrain ahead of us with no semblance of sadness. Like outlining a hiking trail with forking paths and attractive vistas, he detailed the list of pitted molars that could be repaired but would require many fillings and possibly a root canal.

In his mouth, "root" had a neutral sound, like the root of a tree. He didn't linger on it for additional sadistic impact. Yet when he said "root canal," I felt my checkbook with its tiny balance flinch like a salted slug. I hated my teeth, those cold little fuckers with their dramatic displays of pain and histrionic manipulation of my facial nerves. I hated the thought of paying so much money for a tiny and inert piece of chemical and mineral amalgam. Teeth reminded me of the stupid phrase, "Diamonds are a girl's best friend." A diamond is a shitty friend; it just sits there, satisfied with its own price tag, never asking you about your day. The gray of the Boston morning seeped into the room with the prospect of inescapable pain and debt. I winced and asked about the cost. He sighed with sympathy.

"I could pull the worst tooth today for $25," he said. "You'd probably want to get a bridge for the gap eventually, but the pain disappears when the tooth is gone."

Twenty-five dollars was a bargain. He must have made this offer every day to his low-income patients. He was trained to repair teeth, to save them. Instead, he ripped them out, mouth after mouth. But he stopped pain, too, and offered a realistic solution. I imagined patients just like me, who wiped the spit and blood from the corners of their mouths; rubbed their numb jaws; and gathered up their coats, hats, and gloves to face the Boston cold.

I had seen those dark, toothless gaps in Dennis's mouth. He'd taken the direct and affordable route in his teens and twenties when money was needed elsewhere. In his thirties the flesh and skin of his cheeks sunk a few millimeters against the molar-shaped spaces, signaling a wily hunger. If he laughed widely, the dark gaps made him look rakish and daringly snaggletoothed, like the fighter he was. But he dreamt of porcelain bridges. Wherever he is, I know that by now he has paid for those expensive and tiny sculptures. He can remember poverty well enough without needing to touch a daily dental rosary with his tongue.

Twenty-five dollars was a bargain, but the middle-class, orthodon-tized little girl inside me lodged a righteous protest. How, she asked, could I surrender the molars that had so gamely suffered years of expensive orthodontia? What about the headgear, the careful brush-ing, the hooks and rubber bands? To that little girl, pulling a tooth was akin to leaving a kid in foster care so Mommy could go to Foxwoods Casino. It was like selling your Brownie merit badges for crack. It was like giving up on life's promise of better days.

In the three seconds it took me to hear the dentist's price and consider it, I also listened to the little orthodontia girl, who assured me I would eventually get out of this tooth-pulling life. I was not born into it, she said. I came from the land of dental treatment; I believed, if nothing else, that I could choose. Like an antelope rejoining the herd, I could heed my desperation and go corporate, make my escape, and blend into a world of beige partitions and full coverage. So I had to act as if I were already there, in the land of diamonds. My relatives' stories from Arkansas and postwar Ger-many—the times before antibiotics, the times when a cold could lead to death—conjured up dead ancestors who would shame me for coming so close to this healthcare nirvana and turning back from its embrace and its promise.

"Fix them up," I said.

My teeth hurt, and what did that mean? What was my mouth fight-ing for?

If there were an idea to defend through that small dental suffering, it would have to be the idea of stumbling blindly into life without a plan. I could have achieved a complete-dental-benefits package upon graduation, I suppose. I could have got my teaching certificate straight from college. I could have gone back home and worked at my parents' nuclear-safety-licensing business. I could have stayed in the Midwest to apply my skills as a receptionist and thereby burrow into the lowest echelons of a large information industry, such as publishing, and spend a few decades accumulating specialized knowledge about some product I would sell and develop. I could have started college with a clearly defined career path.

Instead, I chose to not know where I was going, and to wander. I left the comforts of networks and family connections to blunder elsewhere alone, and this felt important. But when tested, the strength of my conviction seemed to deaden. It didn't crumble exactly; looking back, I realize I could have gone home to admit defeat, and I never did. But something started to turn in me, as if the pain had nowhere to go but inward. Every pulse of my teeth rang a tinny bell of sadness and resentment, and built up a microscopic accretion of tension in the muscles of my shoulders.

I wanted to look beyond wealth; I thought status symbols were stupid. But the pain created a certain chipped shoulder and weakened version of myself, one that craved comfort in exactly those symbols—a name-brand sweater at Goodwill, a fancy leather purse at a garage sale—as a form of revenge.

Pain is thoughtless. It needs to be mastered and taught, to be given voice. My mute and thoughtless unfixable dental pain burst with a secret suspicion that belied all my ideals. Every metallic ache made me hate myself—either for being physically weak or mentally misguided. Way out near my lips, I could carefully enunciate the words "national healthcare" and the sentence "This system sucks," but those abstract theories were nothing like the sharp insistence of a cracked tooth.

The dentist drew up a game plan. He told me he'd do his best to avoid a root canal, and he was true to his word. The repair required five or six separate visits. "We don't want to hurt you too much at once," he said.

He set to work, and the cold rush of Novocain flooded my gums. The muscles in my shoulders, neck, and head relaxed against the vinyl of the exam chair. I wanted to cry from relief in this naturalist dental paradise of the working class. I shut my eyes and surrendered to the pressure of the worrying drill, engulfed in the sulfurous and woody burning smell of decay disintegrating under the bit. Despite the pain, I enjoyed the austere comfort of fixing a problem, shoring up the foundation.

Over the next few months, my dental visits fell into a weekly routine. Each visit required a $25 co-pay and extra fees for x-rays and fillings. As I sat in the chair during one appointment, I used the vestiges of former mathleticism to add up the fees. Four twenty-fives to a hundred, two, three . . . The total would probably have been enough to pay for one comprehensive visit to a regular dentist.

I took the T to work in the cold that made my face ache. Rattled and shell-shocked from the day's events at the group home, I took the T home at night. I began writing in spiral notebooks to fill every minute of my hour-long commute, writing a novel about everything that I did not have in my life, about a woman artist alone in the rural Midwest. I described the smell of the corn and the dirt and the rain in the sun and called back everything that the gray winter in Boston made me long for. The idea of being a writer seemed, as always, self-indulgent and hardly of service to the revolution—whichever revolution I happened to be signed up for at the time. But I wrote anyway, because Linda had been telling me I needed dreams of my own. There was this thing about building happiness that she wanted me to learn, something about looking in the present for things to savor, not just putting all my hopes in the revolution of someday. At the time, I rationalized my daily writing by telling myself that it kept me from going crazy and therefore kept me of use and in service to the people.

Each week, when I arrived at Linda's office, I flicked on all the lights in the waiting room, which was too large for its present function. A small sofa and two stuffed wingback chairs cowered together in the center of the room around a glass coffee table. The room retained the breathless and nervous energy of hundreds of clients waiting to see their shrinks. The two windows, covered with white venetian blinds, opened on to the airshaft. I embarked once on cleaning these white, plastic slats and found I'd made a grave error. The high ceilings meant that the dirtiest blinds were ten feet in the air. I cleaned the bottom six feet, rattling and smearing dust on the white plastic and finally getting them somewhat clean. But the top four feet of blinds were then disgusting and caked in comparison, and I didn't have a ladder to reach them.

In over my head. What to do? I pulled up a chair, craned my arm skyward.

The tepid sun of early spring trickled through the sludge-flecked window, and the dentist told me to bite to tamp down my last filling. I pressed against a metal wedge that stuffed filling into a live pocket of my skull. He polished off the rough edges, and I left his office in a confluence of small victories: my teeth were fixed. I was new and improved.

I did not exactly notice my teeth. I noticed, instead, that the barometric pressure seemed to be squeezing my sinuses like an aggressive aunt palpating a baby's cheeks. I noticed that the conversation with the gas company about an accidental late fee made me want to hurl the potted coleus through the window. I noticed that a staff meeting gave me a splitting headache. I noticed a subtle layer of defeat blanketing my days. One night—maybe I was sitting at work or leaning back into a hot bath—I took stock of this annoying self-pity and misery, then ran through possible causes. PMS? No, wrong week. Like an idiot, like a dissociated mechanic who has to refer to the owner's manual, I made myself completely still. At once, it became clear—my fucking teeth hurt.

I have since realized (with the help of a cadre of mental health professionals) that my skills in denial are highly developed and might be even considered robust. The pain in my jaw was a dull fog, not a lightning bolt. My mouth, aided by the conniving tongue, shifted food in a constant sideswipe and chewed on the right side only. Several nerve clusters clearly registered alarm; my brain—I realized with embarrassment—had been telling itself for weeks in half whispers that those throbs, those cold shocks, were signs of jaw, teeth, and gums healing, getting back to normal. This committee had to admit the collective defeat of its wishful thinking.

I relented and visited the clinic one last time, almost ashamed at my failure to heal. As I sat in the waiting room, I worried that the dentist would think me a dental hysteric, a needy and soft woman with too many nerve endings. He looked in with his little light, wondering if my fillings were too high. He buzzed at the surface of a molar with his drill bit.

"Bite," he said. He raised his eyebrows expectantly. This was like the eye tests where the optometrist showed me two screens of letters that looked exactly the same. I knew something critical and biological was at stake, and I felt a profound failure in my ability to differentiate.

"Uhhhh . . . yeah, it feels better. Definitely," I said. It was only sore because of the drilling. It was my sinuses. It was the cold. I had a caffeine headache.

As I paid my co-pay and walked home, I fought the realization that my dentist had clearly reached the limits of his dental repertoire. The teeth were bad; the money had been spent; the pain would become background noise, irritating but vaguely ennobling, like a hair shirt. Over the next year, I resigned myself to chewing on the right side of my mouth. The upside was that the pain had morphed from savage and sharp to dull and predictable. At least I had teeth. All I had to do was ask for drinks without ice.

One year later, I quit the group home and got a very, very bad job as the director of a respite home for kids with developmental disabilities such as Down syndrome and autism. The kids were great; the staffers were devoted and fantastic; the administration was a bit flawed. One of our kids had HIV. When I called the main office to request rubber gloves for her diaper changes, the director told me to use sandwich bags. I called the Occupational Health and Safety Administration and left many messages on an answering machine with a recording that sounded like the squawky adult voices in a Charlie Brown cartoon.

Brooke delivered a windfall of good news in the fall of 1996: there was a staff job open at the cool student-organizing nonprofit where she worked as a fundraiser. I put together my application portfolio, the writing clips and list of organizing campaigns, and happily accepted the job after the first applicant turned it down.

At the Center for Campus Organizing, located in the basement of the Old Cambridge Baptist Church, I learned how to use e-mail and was forced to improve my public speaking abilities. Our office featured an inexplicable trapdoor underneath a scrap of carpet that led to a pool of fetid, standing water, and the low ceilings made everyone duck beneath the eaves to get to their desks.

I rode with Mark, the organizer, to a speaking engagement at Yale University. I thought I was going to kill him because he listened to a power-punk medley of Florida bands at top volume, and I prodded him to talk about his God-awful music so he would turn it down. He was quiet, thoughtful, sensitive, and had a great shelf of political books—this time about the civil rights movement and the student movements of the 1960s, which I also knew almost nothing about. He told me about his student-organizing work, and he made me laugh.

I corresponded with student and faculty activists around the country, edited a magazine of campus activism, and got interviewed by the New York Times. Suddenly I was supposed to be an authority on things. Because it was my job, I began to act as if I knew something, seeing in myself the potential to be competent.

Not only was the work challenging and interesting, but I had also won Willie Wonka's golden ticket: real dental. I was a made woman. If I had a dental emergency, I was no longer completely and financially fucked. I ripped open the Delta Dental enrollment package like a birthday present and lovingly ran my fingertips along the rounded edges of the thin, laminated dental card. I sighed with pleasure to behold the group number and member number surrounding my name on the card—each of which corresponded like love letters, like ties of laughter and sweet heartache, to a record in an insurance-claims manager's database. Emboldened and validated, with a newly minted future to protect, I promptly addressed the problem of my molars, because having dental and not using it was like going to a steakhouse buffet and eating a salad, like spitting in the face of fortune.

I lay back on the exam chair in a pale room flooded with fluorescent light and adorned with floral prints in muted pastels, and the smell of that dental office as I remember it brings to mind a feeling of rejoining a comforting hive of the middle class. My benefits package, alas, was far from premium, and half of my treatment costs would stick like leeches to my credit card. But I reasoned that any healthy relationship required meeting one's beloved halfway.

My young, attractive dentist stepped in, exuding the scent of Irish Spring soap from his baby-fresh pores. He picked over my molars one by one with a "hmmm" and a "huh."

"Who did this to you?" he asked.

He explained that the Jet Ski dentist had given me loose fillings; decay had practically been invited to fester along the margin and underside of each pocket and crevice. In effect, my mouth was worse off than if I'd left it alone. Oh, Dr. Outdoorsy Dentist, you tried so hard, but "almost" is not good enough with dental.

Dr. Clean and Fresh scraped away the crust silver, removing all my fillings in order to scrape out the decay that had accumulated underneath. During one of four or five sessions, my jaw froze in the open position and I massaged the joints beneath my ears.

"Close and open your jaws for me," Dr. Clean and Fresh said. I did so with that familiar shimmy of a drawer slid slightly out of its tracks. "Do you hear that clicking? You have TMJ."

Hmmm. Interesting. I shrugged. At that point, adult acronyms mystified me. I thought an IRA and a 401(k) were both accounts you opened if you were interested in buying a large piece of recreational equipment like a yacht. I had no idea what I was supposed to do with the TMJ information, so I considered it as benign a category as my astrological sign. Dr. Clean and Fresh called me afterward to make sure I was okay, and I briefly considered asking him out. I thought for a second I was in love with him, but then I decided that I was infatuated by his ability to heal.

I wanted it to be done. But the teeth still hurt. I couldn't quite get over the grudge I held against the tiny, white devils and couldn't bring myself to approach the intimacy of calling them "mine," so we kept our distance from each other. They poked at me like tiny, peaked, white-cloaked Klan members, snickering with evil when I smiled wrong or when I chewed too hard on Jujubes. They had the power and the element of surprise. They could split and demand an immediate root canal or crown, destroy my small savings in a single swoop.

The body will break, and that's not the hard part. I mind the impermanence less than the thought of being made to pay, to worry about paying, to feel ashamed for being inadequate against the force of those bills, to be beaten by the cost of the inevitable, to have to apologize for the paper version of suffering, which tells me that the cost of living in my body is a price I cannot afford.

The Center for Campus Organizing was run on grants. After we missed a few, Brooke sat for long evening and weekend hours at her desk in the dank basement, staring at the grants database, trying to make money appear. In our dark hours over beer after work, we'd catch glimpses of ourselves from the outside. We were twenty-four and twenty-five. What the hell did we know about running a national nonprofit? To pass the time at work when an international student controversy erupted, we would turn around to each other and sketch out scenes from our imagined reality series, Nonprofit Hell. Brooke began to get sick, too—skin rashes and dizziness among many other problems. We thought maybe she had Lyme disease, and she left work for blood tests that all showed up negative.

Finally, with no money in the account but with a grant check finally in process, we decided to furlough ourselves in December 1997. I got a job at Harvard Bookstore, and one day my friend from college Sharad walked in and plunked a few books down next to my register.

"Hey, Sonya," he said, smiling, the deep voice echoing in his six-foot-plus frame. He had been a good friend of my New York, gangly, smiley, college, anarchist boyfriend; but I had been too intimidated by the epic nature of his presence—all-night pie-making marathons, massive parties, and impromptu drives to North Dakota and back at 120 miles per hour—to spend much time with him. In Boston, off campus and weathered by postcollege life, we listed the friends and dreams of writing we had in common. Sharad invited me over, fed me, and added me to his collection of waifs making illogical decisions. We began to worry about each other back and forth as each of us needed it, which is as good a definition of family as I have found.

Sharad invited Dennis and I over for dinner one night with a group of friends. I arrived and waited for Dennis. We ate a seven-course meal, including some meat that had involved a day or two of elaborate marination and preparation. We drank port. By the time the last chocolate strawberries were eaten, Dennis still had not appeared. Drama ensued; Dennis was located in a bar; and the all-too-familiar pattern earned me a stern talking-to from Sharad, who was concerned about me and my choices.

Brooke worked alone in the office during the furlough without pay, trying to raise money for us. She felt responsible for keeping the place open and got sick from exhaustion. When I returned to work, I started feeling stabbing pains in my guts. The spot of pain I'd joked about for years as my "coffee spot," which ached when I drank more than four large Dunkin' Donuts coffees, seized up my insides one day and I could not breathe or move. I had to have help getting in a cab to the hospital, and the doctors gave me some injection of steroids under the skin, which made no sense to me.

I knew I was falling in love with Mark, but that was more a symptom than a cause of the breakup with Dennis. The socialist-anarchist détente I'd designed in my head as a model of my relationship with Dennis was not sustaining in practice, and politics didn't keep me from feeling lost. Mark was quiet and funny, while Dennis tried to argue me into a corner; I was tired of arguing about politics. I just wanted someone to visit bookstores with. At picket lines for striking UPS workers, Mark yelled as loud as Dennis had. Mark and I had long conversations about the meaning of the student movement, about the next steps for labor.

Brooke and I told each other we needed real jobs. The Center for Campus Organizing moved offices as staff turnover fragmented the organization. Brooke left for New York and law school around the same time that my friend Monica from the group home started law school in Boston. People all around me were acting like adults, or were at least enrolling in graduate programs where they could get their messed-up teeth and bodies temporarily repaired and get a few student loans to rebuild their credit.

With the final funding crisis facing us, I applied for a job in Chicago at a magazine I'd respected for years. I wanted to be their editor; and as is my grateful lot in life, I was their second pick. They offered me a job as an assistant publisher instead, with benefits, for more money than I'd ever made in my life. So in the fall of 1998 Mark and I packed up and moved to the Midwest.

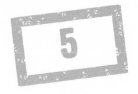

5

FEMALE TROUBLE

On my first day of work at the magazine, the editor pulled me aside and told me the publisher might be leaving and I might be able to have his job. In most fields this offer might be seen as an outrageous stroke of good luck. But within the world of political nonprofits, I had learned that this meant possible trouble ahead. Each day I walked to work and told myself I could handle another day of learning how to make a donor database. I would make five calls to donors and then bribe myself with a break or a cup of coffee. This job was worth it. I was making $25,000, after all, plus benefits! The lower-left molar repaired by Dr. Fresh and Clean cracked, and I had good enough dental that my root canal was halfway covered so it only cost me $1,000.

A nonprofit funding crisis was familiar enough to me that I found ways to survive it for months. To the south of us was Bucktown, a trendy artists' neighborhood in mid-gentrification. To the west was Logan Square, a Latino neighborhood dotted with Mexican bakeries, five-and-dimes, and candy stores. In the summer, we would walk to the El stop and buy mangos on sticks that had been sprinkled with lime juice and chili powder. Pure heaven. We took the El downtown to Blues Fest, to Taste of Chicago, to the lakefront, to the thousands of fantastic street fairs and parades. We had a health plan, so I got to see a psychiatrist and therapist and got back on medication. I felt pretty balanced as far as the panic went. I wrote every morning for an hour and walked to work. I made sure I exercised, and that seemed to make life manageable. I also wrote a few pieces for the magazine and for other outlets, just to keep in touch with the alphabet.

But the money—for a variety of mysterious, nonprofit reasons—was disappearing, and the magazine ran out of money to pay free-lancers. It was my job to tell the staff that the checks for their writers would have to wait.

To distract myself and avert panic, I began to duck out of the office during my lunch breaks. I would buy a Chicago-style hot dog with cucumber, peppers, and tomato from the street vendor and wander the aisles of the amazing thrift store down the street. I loved being back in Chicago, and I drove the hour down to New Lenox on many weekends. I volunteered at a labor community coalition, Chicago Jobs with Justice, and made turnout calls for rallies and pickets. I joined the Logan Square progressive politics association and went to meetings with the Greens and with Chicago labor and independent-media groups. Mark chose to focus on labor issues and stayed home on other nights; now it seems to me that his strategy for sanity was to find nonpolitical outlets like reading and movies, to look for a bit of balance. I might have learned something from him there if I'd been paying attention.

I began to get so nauseous at work that the room tipped. Then I started to get weird pelvic pains. At the time, the doctors asked me if I was under any undue stress; I always scoffed and said, "Nah. I know stress, and this is nothing. You should have seen me last year!"

They tested me for ectopic pregnancy, endometriosis, and pelvic inflammatory disease. The stabbing pains got worse. Somehow with all the blood work, I failed to get a referral for some initial visit from my HMO primary care provider, which started a domino effect of bills. All the charges associated with this mystery condition began to be rejected.

I sat down with the phonebook-sized certificate of benefits from my HMO and with the bills and explanation-of-benefits statements I received in the mail. I started a new manila folder. I took notes on every conversation in order to locate and understand the problem. Basically, I hadn't racked up the right permission within the HMO to see my gynecologist.

No one at the HMO had directed me to the right office or told me what to do. They all worked together within one building, which was supposed to be more efficient; yet they didn't seem to understand how their own organization was supposed to work. I left so many messages with my primary care doctor that she began to actually return my calls. Undoubtedly, I was trying to vent frustration at my own healthcare, my own job situation, onto the shoulders of my HMO, which I figured was a deserving target. I went at it as if it were my job.

Then it was my job. Just as I was scheduled for minor diagnostic surgery so that the doctor could stick a scope in my lower body cavity to see what the hell was going on, our health plan premiums at the magazine shot up tremendously. My boss told me to gather quotes and choose a new health insurance provider. I fielded visits from various plan reps, got heavy cardstock folders filled with detailed plan information. I became overwhelmed. Then I learned that there were services for which you hired a contractor to make these decisions for you. So I fielded quotes from those healthcare-selection contractors, collected their binders and folders, and became once again overwhelmed.

Each contractor who ran the numbers gave us the disturbing picture. We had an older, long-term employee with some major health issues. We had a freelancer working for health insurance. We had a third ex-employee who had settled a dispute with the magazine by receiving health insurance as a settlement. Our overall usage for healthcare put us in a high-premium category.

I was in charge of making sure that all of these people in addition to our regular staff had health insurance. I became so nauseous and addled with pain that I couldn't work. My job consisted of figuring out exactly how little money we made and then calling long-term subscribers and asking them for money. At home Mark and I had halfhearted conversations about the heartbreak of putting our energy into the student movement and then trying to find our way belatedly through post-student life.

Nursing several escape fantasies, I applied for various residencies and grants for writers. The art director at the magazine was also looking for a way out, so I loaned him my grant guide. As he was handing the book back to me, he turned to a page he had bookmarked.

"Did you see this?" he asked.

I scanned the listing that he had pointed to: a fellowship to Ohio State University for midcareer journalists. "No effing way," I said, shaking my head.

"I think you should apply for it," he said. He looked at me, and the emphatic way he said it made me feel a little guilty for dismissing him so lightly. Maybe he would think I wasn't grateful.

"Okay," I said, and I spent the next few weeks putting together my writing clips and my essay.

As the cutting cold of the Chicago winter turned to spring, I found a health plan for the magazine and had my surgery, which revealed fluid in my pelvis that was probably the result of a previous infection. I also won a grievance case against my HMO, and the benefits office was required to send out a mailing to every female in the network to clearly explain the plan's reproductive-health benefits. These victories felt so very, very unsatisfying. Sometimes I sit with my head in my hands and think about all the hours lost. I could have been learning Spanish. I could have been learning to play the saxophone.

I decided I had to get out of the magazine. Done. That was it. I'd rather clean houses, I told my mom. She agreed and said there was good money to be made. As I designed my house-cleaning-service business cards, I gave my notice at the magazine. I applied for as many clerical jobs as I could find and considered going into a sheet metal apprenticeship. After the first orientation training at the Women in the Building Trades office, I got a call from Ohio State, and the program director said he wanted to interview me. I got a summer job as a secretary at a church, had my interview, and was accepted into the journalism program at OSU. In other words: healthcare and paid grad school.

Mark moved with me from Chicago to Columbus in the summer of 1999, though by this time we had dug out opposing sides in a staring contest that would lead to nowhere good. We went on a summer-long road trip that involved a whole vanload of awkward silences. We moved our stuff from a storage unit to an apartment, and then capped off the grueling move with a breakup.

That fall, I tried to listen to the chorus of therapists and stay single. But within a few months I met my next boyfriend, Skate. He was a carpenter and an artist. I figured my problem had been in dating organizers, so I decided to try a completely different approach. Plus, Skate could build a bookshelf, cook a meal in a crock-pot, and fix a toilet: a DIY boyfriend.

I chose the issue of workplace safety in the mental health industry for my journalism thesis project and began interviewing direct care workers and union reps. I started working with a socialist labor group in Detroit, so I drove from Columbus on weekends for labor conferences and then crashed afterward with my friend Sharad, who was living at his parents' house. His dad kindly listened to my socialist rants and told me about his stint with socialism in India, and his mom packed me tins of outstanding homemade Indian food for the drive home. Sharad didn't care that I was a socialist. "I can feed you and then I don't have to donate to any official causes. You do that all for me," he said, laughing. "My little commie."

Like a charming cousin with a cocaine addiction, my body was always getting me into expensive trouble. I was already a case file for a medical collections agency. The manila folder labeled "Health Insurance Hell" I started in Chicago had grown larger and now contained records from an awesomely named collections agency, the Medical Bureau of Economics. Because a doctor in Boston in 1997 had failed to submit a referral form for a minor outpatient procedure, even though I'd asked her three times to do so, I got stuck with a $75 charge. I disputed it, didn't hear anything, and then moved from Boston to Chicago to Columbus. MBE found me and let me know that $75 had mysteriously morphed into a $383.15 debt. In graduate school $75 was quite a lot of money, and $383.15 was rent. MBE assigned a collections person to my case, and he would leave messages like, "This is Neil. We need to talk."

When we spoke, Neil addressed me with restrained sarcasm, as if I'd charged a plasma-screen television and then flaked on the payments. He needled; he threatened to garnish my paycheck; and he called me at work, at inappropriate hours of the evening, and in the early morning. I wrote letters with bullet points, outlining the chronology of my treatment and the charges, listing every possible account number and doctor's name, trying to convince him that this amount was not my responsibility. Neil was not moved by my suggestion of a payment plan, and he was not moved by slobbering pleas for mercy or by temper tantrums of by rage. If anything, he seemed to lose respect for me.

I asked my mom for advice. She said she had heard that if a

collections agency cashed a check bearing the words "Paid in Full" on the memo line, it couldn't dispute the payment later in court. This sounded like using a horoscope as a binding legal contract, but I was desperate. I made out a check for $75 and wrote "Paid in Full" on the memo line. For some reason known only to large buildings, Neil disappeared from my life.

Over the coming years, I would begin to hyperventilate at the sight of an explanation of benefits issued by an insurance agency. I would learn to call 1-800 numbers and challenge claims evaluators on their coding of medical procedures, saving hundreds of dollars every year. I would take such battles to my insurer, my state attorney general, and my insurance company's patient mediation board. In my subsequent correspondence, I would mention the previous correspondence and use the words "subsequent," "previous," and "correspondence."

That spring of 2000, as I delved into the last part of my coursework, the housekeeping and maintenance staff at Ohio State ran into negotiation difficulties with the university administration and prepared to go on strike. So I hung out at the meetings and on the picket lines. The student labor coalition took over the administration building to pressure the university to bargain with the union, so I spent the night in a sleeping bag on the linoleum outside the president's office.

A few days after my labor sleepover, Sharad and two of his buddies drove down from Detroit to visit. They stumbled from a twelve-foot-high SUV in a piñata-like explosion of fast-food wrappers, clove-cigarette smoke, and empty CD cases. Sharad and the boys bought lots of beer and stayed up watching kung fu movies at top volume. I fled to Skate's house at 2 a.m. The next morning, after coffee, I went home to greet Sharad and the boys, who ate breakfast, broke a chair, and started drinking again. Then they watched more kung fu, and finally I had to ask them to leave.

Lack of sleep and water, combined with too much sex and coffee, led me into the borderland between sick and well. My joints began to ache. Where the hell were my kidneys, anyway? Kidneys had to be near my hips, not way up near my shoulder blades. Putting them so high up would obviously be a design flaw. So if that ache wasn't my kidneys (clearly not), it must be the kind of healthy ache one gets from exertion and recovery, the signal of a crisis averted, the recharged body bouncing back from a near miss. Yeah. I was young, wiry, and flexible, a pickup-truck-driving midwestern girl with a ponytail and strong hands. I could cure a sinus infection with a pint of beer, a fever with a clove of raw garlic. I was twenty-eight, a good girl who was careful never to bounce checks but who also occasionally found herself down to a can of black olives in the pantry, making toast and olives for dinner.

I was getting a little run-down, and as usual I was having trouble prioritizing and getting sleep because everything seemed so important. I slurped cranberry juice in my rented kitchen. I was two days away from a long-scheduled research trip in Chicago that would lead to the end of graduate school. But whatever. What mattered was that this was the sprint, the final leg, the dash to the finish line that drew from marathon runners the hidden reserves to power themselves along.

The stupefaction of fever allowed me to conclude that driving and writing were both sitting, so nearly lying down, so nearly the same as lying in bed. Using the same logic as countless ex-boyfriends who staggered to work and to the bar while harboring bronchitis and strep throat and disturbingly infected wounds and chronic migraines, I decided to show my body and some stupid teeny bacteria who was boss. Maybe if I had been uninsured at that moment, I would have known I was playing with my life. But because I had the bounty of the student health card in my wallet, I figured that, for once, my healthcare was under my control. That sounds logical, I guess, maybe even sociological.

And yet there is a yellow aura of sickly mania around my memories from these days, a nephrologic pushing and desperation to get the impossible done, the knowledge that after the summer, I would be booted from graduate school, planless. The linoleum in the grimy kitchen peeled. I had no plan. A hole in the wall sprouted wires from a phone ripped out by a previous tenant's tantrum. I had a thousand résumés and a thousand envelopes. I had no plan. The world was spread before me like a busload of Czechoslovakian stamp collectors asking the way to the convention hall in a language I did not speak.

I hunched over a shopping cart filled with two plastic two-liter bottles of store-brand cranberry juice cocktail. I took a slow and curative breath in to dissipate pain that radiated from my groin to my armpits. I knew I had a urinary tract infection, the "honeymoon malady," the most common infection in the human body, the infection that accounts for more than eight million doctors' visits a year in the United States. If you have not had one, imagine peeing Tabasco for a week straight.

With my cranberry juice riding shotgun, I kissed Skate good-bye and headed west on I-70, blasting music and cold air, forcing sickness from my body with bracing draughts of road-trip, blue-sky joy. The six-hour drive from Columbus to Chicago took eight with bathroom breaks. In my triumphant victory over infection, I happily stopped at gas stations to climb out of my red pickup truck and feel the gravel under my boots. I blinked against a haze in my vision and turned up the radio, keeping a finger on the radio's Seek button and finding one Led Zeppelin song after another. In my complicated hybrid of classic rock and tarot, Zep on the radio signaled good luck and benevolence ahead—handy and affirming in the rural Midwest, which is enveloped like a force field in the song "Stairway to Heaven." Under the favorable constellation of Zep, my little red truck buzzed farther and farther beyond the boundaries of my health plan's network of approved providers. The flatland of Illinois fanned out like a warm and welcoming pancake, the land that I love.

I reached my parents' house and my old room, and all the past recoveries from various mental and physical ailments seemed to be cheering me on from the bench. "It's nothing! You're a star!" roared mononucleosis and chicken pox from the sidelines. "Now get to work!"

I bent to grab a stack of notebooks. Pain shot around my torso to my sternum, and my scalp was soaked with beads of sweat. "Argh," I muttered, releasing sickness with my groan. I was now apparently a certified new age self-healer. I mumbled, "Testing, testing," into the tape recorder between gulps of lukewarm cranberry juice. That ache was certainly not my internal organs.

I went down to the kitchen for more juice and for assistance in building my fortress of denial. "Wow, I'm really sore," I said to my mom. "I think I'm getting over something. Does that ever happen to you?"

As luck would have it, she was recovering from bronchitis. Her chest muscles, she said, had been sore for a week.

See? There you go.

The narrative cure—telling stories to heal—was also advocated by Brenda Ueland, Minnesotan author of the 1920s writers' classic *If You Want to Write*. The book relates chapters of enthusiastic and invigorating writers' advice infused with a pioneer can-do spirit. She also relates an anecdote about a violinist who cured a fever by staying up all night playing rapid, sawing trills on her instrument. I'm too much of a wuss to write poetry through a sinus infection, but I envy the ability to blast a horde of viruses from the bloodstream with a to-do list and the healthy surge of production. And the research trip to Chicago was productive, but the most important lesson I learned was this: if pee fizzes like soda pop, it's time to find the ER.

I drove north from my parents' house to downtown Chicago for a day of research. I visited three mental health facilities, gathered reports and interviews, and stopped at a federal agency to file forms requesting figures on occupational health and safety. Fever continued as a backdrop to the paperwork. Tiny electric tracers speckled in my peripheral vision—yellow and purple dots in the gray March sky.

In an afternoon gap between appointments, I drove to a parking garage near a movie theater, turned off the car, and rested my head on the steering wheel. My thoughts seemed to creep by like trundling boxcars. In the spaces between each thought, I saw daylight and nothing else. Combining Brenda Ueland's art cure and my friend Sharad's kung fu movie recommendations, I bought a ticket to a John Wu movie. The blurred dances of whirling feet and glinting swords did not restore me. I sat in the back row of the darkened theater and bent my limbs into the folds of my body like a potato bug, shuddering against the edges of delirium.

My evening schedule included dinner with my ex, Mark, who had moved back to Chicago after our breakup. I'd wronged him on repeated occasions, and we'd scheduled a meal to finally sit down and discuss our demised relationship like two adults. We arranged to meet at a bus station, and I pulled up to the curb to collect him. He slammed the door and settled in, turning to me to hear news about the last year of my life, eyes expectant with the hope for sanity and friendly release of bygone days that the formerly engaged must show toward each other.

I started to cry. "I can't do this," I blubbered. "I'm sick, something is wrong. Something is wrong, I have to leave."

His forehead creased in concern. "I'll help. Where do you need to go?"

"I have to go to the hospital. I have to leave." With my hair sticking out like a Chia Pet and tears and snot streaking down my face and my glasses, I dropped him off at another corner.

Blinding red brake lights swirled. Heat came from inside me, and I knew, finally, that this was bad. I turned the truck south into rush-hour traffic on the ominously beautiful Dan Ryan Expressway. A mysterious jumble of wooden scaffolding and gnarled machines squeezed traffic at the shoulders into gathers and shirred ripples of a bottleneck, curving under viaducts and down massive concrete channels like cells of contagion in a glowing blood vessel. I called my mom. I called Skate in Ohio. "Something is wrong," I said. I cried in the bumper-to-bumper traffic and set my fingernails against the maroon plastic of the steering wheel.

"Try to sleep," said my mom, putting me in bed. "If you still feel bad in the morning, we'll go to the ER."

At midnight I woke up in a dry heat with an urgent, metallic sensation soaking my skull. I stood and the room pitched. In the dark I trailed my hands along the wall toward my parents' room, wondering wordlessly like a five-year-old whether it was urgent enough to wake my mom. That downbeat—two, three—as I listened to Mom breathe and Dad snore and watched Mom's pink fingers, flung across the covers, twitching. Felt guilt about interrupting a dream. I was being silly. Fevers passed. That's what they did, and sleep cured all. I sighed against the froth in my head.

"Mom. I think we need to go now," I whispered. "I'm not right." Her eyes opened and focused so quickly that they seemed to reach back a few seconds in time to make up for the dream state, to gather the force needed to be a mother in the middle of the night.

We drove under the black sky to the hospital, the same place I'd volunteered in high school as a candy striper in a white and red–striped ruffled smock. Growing up, I'd listened to people from church, friends of my parents, laugh and trade stories about mistakes made by doctors, the wrong leg amputated. But I felt safe in the waiting area, muffled with normal noise of midnight television. Soon they would give me drugs, and I would mend and get on with my life. Instead, they pointed to a cot and handed me a paper gown.

"It's freezing in here," I shuddered. "Can I have a blanket?"

The nurse turned down her mouth. "No. You feel cold because your fever is 105 degrees."

My grandmother, Elfriede Klejdzinski, died at age forty-seven in Germany after World War II. A kidney infection—probably caused by a UTI—killed her. Thankfully, my mom and I didn't know this on the night of my ER trip. We figured it out years later during a family research project, with the help of Elfriede's death certificate. Mom tells me the whole German family blamed my grandfather for not taking my grandmother to the hospital soon enough.

He told his wife to rest and see if she felt better in the morning. Then, I imagine, the curtain of fever descended. I don't think she said good-bye to her children. My mother was six, and her brothers were nine and four. It must have seemed like routine female trouble, a simple ailment. Chaos, caused by the assumption or hope that the body could cure itself, rippled outward from that bit of bacteria.

The nurses gave me a room and a bed. I felt splattered and disjointed like a microwaved Jackson Pollock painting. I kept asking the nurses if I was going to die. They patted my arm and told me the fever was a sign that my body was fighting the infection. But then I overheard them standing in the hall at shift change, saying to each other, "It's still at 105," with muted frustration. They took my temperature every hour and clipped massive bags of antibiotics and antifebrile medicine to the IV pole.

My mother and I argued.

"Call the nurse," I said. "I feel really crappy. My fever's up again." I knew this because words would not connect in my head. They repelled one another like magnets turned the wrong way, refusing links to make meaning. I couldn't remember how to worry, couldn't tell myself any internal story. I was just a body gone awry, and the flavor of my personality was a taste I couldn't recall.

"It couldn't be up. They just gave you Motrin." Mom wanted me better. I pressed the call button; the nurse came, took my temperature, and sighed. Yes, it was up. I glared at my mom: *See, you are a terrible mother. You want me to die!*

The nurses put ice packs under my armpits and at the back of my neck. When the fever stayed up, they wheeled in a huge machine that pumped chilled water through a plastic blanket. I rolled onto the blanket and winced. The cold made my skin sting and my bones ache. "It's better than an ice bath," said one nurse. "And that's next."

The doctors came in and asked me to explain myself. "We don't understand how a healthy woman would get a UTI this bad. Why did you not go to the clinic earlier? This infection is in your kidneys. If it goes into your blood, there is nothing we can do."

My parents and my brother and sister-in-law and sister crammed into the little room. They told all the family near-death experiences we normally don't talk about. We laughed hysterically about each one—or at least I did. My brother told me his story about getting a 105.7-degree fever in college. The nurses tried to put him in ice, and he told them to fuck off and he left. So funny! And the framed print opposite my bed, the one of the purple flower, was so, so beautiful. And the Jell-O, the lovely green Jell-O, was so, so pure and clear and good.

On the third day, my fever crept down below triple digits and stayed there.

"You look better," said my mom, her face creased and washed out with exhaustion. She had stayed by my bed all night, dozing on and off in the chair.

"Yeah, yesterday your skin was gray. You've got some color," said my dad. I shuffled into the bathroom, dragging the IV stand. I looked

like a corpse, my skin the weird yellow gray of a pre-tornado sky. My
fingers itched for a pen and a legal pad. Praise the Lord, I needed to
make a to-do list. Top priority, now that I would live, was the need
to deal with the potentially catastrophic price tag of a three-day
hospital stay . . . out of network.

I called the 1-800 number for my student health insurance. The
claims agent asked a few basic questions but seemed eager to get
off the phone. I asked in as many ways as I could think of, "Will anything bad happen to me now?" But it came out as, "Is there anything
else you need from me?" What I meant was, will I be punished? Is
the scary part about to begin, now that I'm back at the edges of
normal life?

I wanted the insurance company to share my joy at health restored.
I wanted to throw an alive-again party with a piñata and candy and
fruity drinks. I had not ever been that close to death. The bacteria
had surged and been beaten back with the blessed, lovely panacea
of modern technology. "I do regret my echinacea, earth-first days,"
I muttered. I do love pharmaceuticals. Without the assistance of
our amped-up and hyperfunded-medical-research system, I would
have been a bug splattered on the windshield. I vowed never to
criticize healthcare again, because it had given me life. I promised
myself I would gratefully write checks in whatever amounts were
demanded of me.

The next morning, the doctor arrived to set me free. He sat down
on my bed and studied my chart, reviewing the victory of my clear
blood tests. My mother smiled at him. My sister got up to shove my
belongings into plastic patient-property bags.

"So you're in college," said the doctor, in a mysterious Eastern
European accent. "We need you to avoid any more UTIs. I want you
to do these things: First, try to avoid hot tubs. There are a lot of
bacteria in there. Have you been to any hot tub parties? I know that's
a popular thing in college these days."

I shook my head no. It was a waste of time to describe the wide chasm of behavior, resources, and angst separating graduate students from hot tub parties.

He looked back down at the chart. "Have you been having anal sex?" he asked good-naturedly. My sister spluttered, and my mother's eyes seemed to detach from her mind, as if she were going to wait this one out somewhere far away.

"No," I said.

He nodded. "Well, if you do, you know that you want to avoid the combination of anal and vaginal sex unless you wash very carefully. Veeeery carefully." Mom nodded as if she were receiving instructions about caring for a houseplant or receiving penance.

"Finally, remember to pee after sex. Mmm-kay? Every time," he said. He snapped closed the metal cover of my chart, shook my hand, and wished me luck with my urethra.

My boyfriend Skate called from Ohio for the update. My sister handed me the phone and said loudly, delighting in the one-liner she received from heaven like a treasure, "You can have phone sex, but remember to pee when you're done."

I gingerly drove back to Ohio. I rested. I was a reformed body in gentle communion with her immune system. Who's boss? No, not I. The organs, yes sir, yes ma'am. I drank cranberry juice and dipped my toes into the swirling current of graduate school. I also took my first two creative-writing workshops and soon had to plan on hours of insomnia after those night classes. The pent-up years of desire to write and the collection of writing I'd done in solitude finally had a target, and the energy seemed to explode from me after each workshop.

Weeks into the spring quarter, the first bill arrived. Brave and solemn, I sat down on my couch, determined to take this like a needle-stick, like a good and grateful patient. The itemized charges filled two pages, and each figure was calculated to a specific and seemingly prime number, like $167.49. Each amount was imaginary. I studied the piece of paper as if watching the first flourishes of a ritualized form of warfare from an unfamiliar culture.

These symbolic implements—the dollar signs with their fierce threats—promised damage on the heels of healing. But I had faith in my prearranged, voodoo garlic necklace, the insurance agency, which I hoped would reply with an equally mysterious show of force. I was now drawn into the epilogue of healing, the forced expression of my gratitude with money I did not have.

The salvo was met with a response. "This Is Not a Bill," announced a bill-like statement from the insurance agency. This explanation of benefits promised to clarify things. The gesture was multilayered, with a shift of alliances I could not decipher, a column of codes for benefits' determinants and curt phrases explaining denial of coverage, reduced percentages, and fees for services rendered. I thought I'd paid the insurance agency for its friendship and loy-alty, but apparently I had not paid it adequate homage. The insur-ance agency and the hospital, both large buildings, appeared to have a long-standing relationship cemented with secret winks and handshakes. They whispered strings of codes in a foreign tongue, a conversation I was unable to interrupt.

Other statements appeared. I came to recognize them because they did not need to clarify their intentions. They *were* bills, demand-ing, "Tear Off and Remit." I cried whenever the mailman dropped letters through the slot. After the honeymoon of healing wore off, I was immobilized with financial guilt and fear triggered by the sight of my name in a modernistic, sans-serif font in all capital letters, glaring through the plastic window of an unadorned envelope.

I have never visited a prostitute, but I imagine an itemized bill listing the cost of each ear lick ($0.89) and thrust ($4.03) would be a bit degrading. Similarly, the itemized bill from my near-death experience listing each blood test and kidney ultrasound seemed wrong on a gut level. It was either a bit too much information or not enough. It's not that I didn't want to pay the cost of health. I am cheap, but my cheapness is not the point. I would have cooked a roasted chicken with lemon, dill, and rice pilaf for the blood technician or the night nurse who helped to heal me. And I do not cook. And I am not overly nice. I don't believe in heaven or in doing random acts of kindness to score points on the God pinball machine. The universe mandates gratitude for one's life.

There was—is—something holy and inscrutable about holding the pale, bare crook of one's arm out for a needle. Awareness narrows to a point of hope the size of a pinprick. Take this liquid and prove me well. When the blood technician visited me with her tray of vials during my hospital stay, I felt relief in the sense of a possible narrative turning point, the opportunity to produce and show I was worthy to cross into health. The plastic tubes glugged full with dark red blood, colored caps for each different test, plastic stickers bearing my name. The blood tech joked about my nice veins, told me how tattooed tough guys and heroin addicts were the biggest babies when it came to getting stuck with needles.

I sat with my hospital bills and wished I could directly pay those nurses and blood technicians. I would gladly pay for health itself and for the care that delivered this health. But the nurses received the same amount per twelve-hour, bloody, and heartbreaking shift whether or not they were kind, whether or not they joked with me. The blood tech did not get paid by the vial, but the hospital did.

My involvement with the strike on campus led me to wonder why there wasn't a Jobs with Justice chapter in the city. I met with a few labor organizers I'd met while doing strike support and figured I'd start the local group.

Before the end of the school year, the student labor group

organized a vanload of custodial workers and students to head out to the national Jobs with Justice conference in Boston. The conference involved too much beer and a few temporarily missing custodial workers, whom we found semidrunk at Wal-Mart.

I attended a workshop on single-payer healthcare and shook my head at the history of the healthcare movement offered in bullet points on the blackboard. "We lost the public debate," said one speaker, "because nobody knows what 'single-payer' means. It's jargon." "Amen," I wanted to say.

At a break in the workshop, I chatted with a few organizers near me who happened to work for a healthcare nonprofit in Ohio. "We're looking for a Columbus organizer," one of them said. "It sounds like you have a lot of local contacts."

The next day, after rousing rallies and speeches from labor organizers from Korea and Brazil and lots of yelling and chanting in multiple languages I did not speak, I ran into one of my old college friends, J—— the anarchist, who was doing labor work as an organizer in Vermont and who also knew my friends in the Chicago labor movement. "Let's go for a walk," he said, characteristically wise and still. "I need to get away from all this craziness."

We walked through the tall pines on a trail near the edge of campus, and he told me he craved time off from organizing. We surveyed our political careers in the ten years since we'd started college, charting our shared ups and downs. I asked him what he thought about me going back into organizing and told him there was a healthcare-organizing job in Columbus.

"I thought you just told me you were starting the Columbus Jobs with Justice chapter." He studied me with blue eyes, his lips slightly pursed as he considered me. "Don't get burned out," he said. "You don't have to do this your whole life."

At the time I was an apprentice in the healthcare-insurance ninja adventure. I knew some of the tricks. But when the truckload of kidney-infection bills arrived, I was clueless, utterly unaware of the magic spells and hexes that might have delivered me to safety. I added the figures and found that I owed a tenth of my gross income. But how could I complain? I had to admit that $2,000 was a great deal for getting to see the rest of one's life. Besides, the whole infection thing had been my fault. And this time, I could not blame a forgetful doctor or a paperwork snafu. I'd strayed from my network into the wilds of self-payer land.

Abusive relationships are sometimes characterized by a disturbing process called "traumatic bonding," in which someone threatens you with injury or death. After the meanie utters this threat, he or she is filled with remorse and acts nice. The abused feels saved and hopeful that she will never have to feel so scared again. She becomes grateful to this mean person for not being mean all the time, so she loves the meanie even more deeply for the nice moments. Then the meanie gets grouchy and threatens her life again. In terror she hopes for the nice version to emerge; when it does, she is soooo grateful and tries to figure out what she can do to never make the person mad again.

This cycle of abuse reminds me of my relationship with medical-billing employees and insurance cards. They are too powerful to hate. They usher me through the gates of healing, into health and the rest of my life. They relieve pain and then they whack the shit out of me. I spend so much time learning to be assertive and state my needs in this relationship, as if the relationship itself could ever be healthy or based on mutual respect and open communication. Instead, what I should have done was maybe to leave and go far, far away to somewhere safe, like Sweden or Canada.

After stretching my checkbook to the limit paying my bills in the early summer of 2000, I sat on my living room floor and cried. I was just about done with graduate school, on the fruitless search for a job at a daily newspaper. I could not afford COBRA coverage when my student health coverage ran out, and I certainly could not meet my hospital payments. I called the hospital in tears, and a billing clerk sighed. Kindly, she said, "You know, we can put you on a payment plan."

I stopped crying. "Are you serious?" I said. "Yes, please!" I laughed.

She explained that I could set a reasonable amount to send in each month and that, as long as I was making those payments, my account wouldn't be sent to collections.

That summer, as I looked for work and freelanced and finished my degree, I paid the full $2,000. I did not know that if I had read the back of the tiny gray print on the hospital bill, I could have applied for a low-income fee waiver. The hospital would have written off the debt as part of its social duty to help the poor and would even have gotten a tax break. And I would have had to pay nothing.

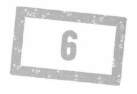

6

HEALTHCARE FOR ALL, ALMOST

One evening on campus in July 2000 as graduation loomed, I ate cubed cheese from a fancy snack tray and swilled pink wine from a plastic cup, pretending to celebrate my hypothetical leap into career security. The tenth person at the graduation reception asked me about my career plans in the field of journalism. I averted my eyes to stare at the doomed sacrificial kale on the cheese tray and felt a pang of sympathy.

I wanted to say, "Oh, I'll be starting with the *New York Times* as their Pacific Rim correspondent."

Lacking daily newspaper experience, I'd been rejected by the likes of the *East Wilmington Bi-Weekly Stenograph and Telegraph* in rural Ohio. My résumé bristled with social-justice verbiage and nonprofit work, but I vowed to give it a haircut and clean it up good. I would work anywhere normal, I promised myself, anywhere with stability and health insurance. I would become someone who wore pleated khakis. Two versions of me diverged in a wood, and I . . . I clearly needed medication.

Either I did cry next to the cheese tray at that reception or I cried in the bathroom or I saved it for the walk home from campus. I know I stumbled up the sidewalk toward my apartment with my face stinging. I cried in chopped coughs from the back of my throat—that "ah-ah-ah" little-kid asthma sound. I gave myself a crying headache, cried so hard I saw violet spots behind my eyelids.

No phone messages, no messages, no messages. Like a watched pot that never boiled, the voice mails from prospective employers evaporated the second I keyed in my access code. I could have started a national search for journalism jobs, but I had a boyfriend, Skate, already in Columbus and made the decision to stay in town. I tweaked my cover letter to emphasize my proficiency with the suite of Microsoft Office applications but couldn't get a callback for an administrative position, never mind a reporting job.

After collecting my diploma, I wadded up the sweaty mess of my black polyester gown and cried some more. I wrapped myself in a frantic whisper: what now, what now? I turned tail and slunk back to the land I knew. The nonprofit version of my résumé burst through its weak and spindly office cousin, glad to be back in command.

I had received the job ad for organizer of the Universal Health Care Action Network at the Jobs with Justice conference that spring, and I'd taken it home and tacked it to a bulletin board near my desk. The Universal Health Care Action Network wins my award for the best acronym ever—UHCAN, as in "You Can!"—which I love for its ungainly and earnest policy recommendation masked with a poetic and emphatic assertion that we could accomplish the impossible.

Each day as I contemplated the journalism job ads online, I saw that ad in the background. There was a certain comfort in using skills I knew I had. I also wanted to hear the applause in my head for doing "good," thereby assuaging the guilt I felt at merely living with all my privileges and advantages. I don't think the latter motive impels most social-justice organizers, but the former—seeking the familiar—strikes many of us, regardless of profession. I chose what I knew, and I knew what I was getting into. I dropped the envelope to UHCAN in the mailbox, and a familiar nudge poked from between my ribs. I'd traded one kind of fear for another.

Cathy, UHCAN's policy director, was a five-foot-zero, laser-focused, healthcare-policy savant. She impatiently pushed back a frizz of orange hair as she described the problems faced by Latino immigrants at one of local the emergency rooms. Interested? Of course I was, I replied. And as for the job itself . . . ? Full time, she said, but no benefits.

"You know the situation, obviously," she said, with a wry and pained smirk. "Small nonprofits can't afford it." Her husband, a surgeon at the local children's hospital, had great benefits. She lived with healthcare. She got to make love to healthcare. She reproduced with healthcare and had healthcare's children.

I balked. "I really need insurance," I said.

"Maybe we can figure something out," she said.

I shook her hand and smiled with bright confidence—I knew I'd get the job. Organizing was all I'd done, and I was probably overqualified. As I pulled away from the church that housed the UHCAN office, however, a gray queasiness spread from my stomach. I imagined the creased and worried faces of all of my past, hardworking therapists. They nickered and shook their carefully styled heads: "Sonya, Sonya, Sonya. When are you going to start taking care of yourself? If you don't do it, no one else will." I accelerated into traffic in a bit of a rage. Screw you, chorus of therapists.

My task was to build a network of the uninsured and raise money and awareness about access to healthcare. My commitment to the position was infinitesimal, ephemeral—a few months of frustration in that upstairs office of the church in eastside Columbus. I find myself still cashing in constantly on what I learned there. At the time, I focused on the downsides: the job made me want to kill myself and I did not receive health insurance.

What follows are a few sample days, an hors d'oeuvres tray of grassroots healthcare reform, compiled from snippets of desperate memory and bitter one-liners in my journals. I did not know then that all was not lost; a full-time reporting position awaited me in the fall. And as it turned out, I would use every single trick I learned at UHCAN on my own healthcare debacles.

I unlocked the heavy front door of the African Methodist Episcopal Mt. Zion Church on Columbus's east side. Shuffling along the gray overwaxed linoleum, I passed the church office and the hallway that lead to BREAD (Building Respect, Equality, and Dignity), a coalition of religious groups channeling the most powerful voice for social justice in Columbus. The BREAD office exuded the buzz of manic activity, a by-product of the hard-line and often-confrontational strategies and direct actions launched against real estate redlining and slumlords. Cathy had counseled me to use BREAD's organizing strategy to build a healthcare network.

I walked through a rectangle of golden light, reflected from a window of rippled yellow glass high up in the stairwell. The stairwell smelled like the cinder block annex of St. Jude's Church from my childhood—an aroma of simple purpose, dank cement, white candles, floor wax, and industrial paint. I wanted to embody that smell, to go about my work with the focus and patience of a nun, with simple and calm attention to first one task, then the next. Alas, that mode of existence would have required constant contact with a benevolent, superhuman presence. Instead of that communion, I had a spiritual hole into which I poured caffeine and a craving for immediate and external approval.

I lacked faith in my work. I believed in immediate constraints and fixtures. For example, I had faith that my boss's desk did indeed exist underneath the sloping wave of policy reports. Another cresting and falling swell of documents lined the baseboard along the left wall of our one-room office, as if to mark the space for an imaginary bookshelf. A cardboard box of brochures, "Where to Get Free Healthcare," angled like a lifeboat in the paper sea. The brackish standing pools of information held no implicit promise of clear sailing toward victory.

My desk sat against the right-hand wall, as lonely as the rectangular corral for a newly hired telemarketer. I did not have a computer. Pink "While You Were Out" memos with curled edges and coffee stains lay in stacks on the desk's faux-wood-grain surface. It seemed to take too much effort to adorn my desk with a mug for pens. The idea of bringing in a framed photo overwhelmed me.

Cathy whirled into the office and flung her briefcase onto the floor. She nodded hello to me, cell phone clutched between shoulder and ear as she plunged both hands into the papers on her desk.

"What do you mean, the amendment hasn't been added?" she demanded to her anonymous conversational partner. She located a folder, stuffed it into her briefcase, and sighed, stopping to roll her eyes. "Yeah, I'll be there at ten. I'm running late."

She clicked the phone closed and faced me. I had stopped to watch her. She watched me back, eyebrows up. "What's going on?" she asked, implicitly wondering why I would waste three seconds of the healthcare battle.

"I organized the filing system," I said, pointing to the metal cabinet.

"Okay," she said. "What are you doing today?"

"Umm," I said, "maybe we can talk tomorrow about goals and stuff like that."

"You're the organizer. Figure out an organizing strategy, and make a work plan," she said, tightening her lips around her teeth. "We can do whatever you want. I have to get to this hearing at the statehouse."

She shut the door. Her steps echoed down the stairwell. As the noise receded, the muscles in my neck and back slowly slackened. I took a few breaths, enjoying the silence. Calm seemed to spread outward from my body, until it ran up against the policy documents surrounding me on all sides.

This was my job. It was a good job. In how many jobs can you do whatever you want? I took out a legal pad and stared at the bleached blue void. So . . . universal healthcare. Hmmmm. To do.

A few days later, I asked Cathy about health insurance.

She sighed. "Call the national office in Cleveland, and see if they can add you to their plan."

The manager at the national office in Cleveland called a benefits consultant, and it turned out that my age and my uterus made me an insurance liability. I might decide to procreate at any moment, I supposed, just to test the ceiling on my stress level. The executive director in Cleveland suggested I purchase an individual policy, and the office would pay part of the fee.

I shivered with a dread as dry as a box of manila folders. This wasn't the first time an employer had asked me to create and propose my own healthcare solution. The task is best left to someone with training in human resources and contract negotiation, someone who has months to gather information and weigh the options.

For me, each of those months was filled with about thirty uninsured days. I studied my COBRA policy from the university, which offered me the option to buy a few months of additional healthcare for an exorbitant fee. A cobra is a venomous, slippery, fanged reptile. In all capital letters, the cruel acronym seems to imply a 1970s movie starring Chuck Norris: COBRA!

I declined to wrestle the cobra and instead collected shiny enrollment packets from three or four companies. Doctors in stock photos waved stethoscopes and smiled. For $300 a month, I could get a $1,000 deductible and 50 percent coverage for catastrophes. Is the glass half full or half empty? Are you a woman or a mouse? I wrote up a list of prices for the national office and tried to think healthy thoughts. My chorus of past therapists sighed and went out for cigarettes.

One of my daily tasks at UHCAN was to check the "healthcare hotline," a voice-mail line for collecting the stories of people on the edge of medical and financial chaos. We took notes from these messages and then counseled callers to help sort through their hospital bills.

I keyed in the access code. A midwestern, male voice, polite and measured, told the story of his former employer, which had declared bankruptcy and would not pay his guaranteed retiree benefits. He didn't have money for a lawyer and didn't know what to do with the stack of bills for his kidney dialysis and medications. He gave a quiet, bemused half chuckle and asked for any help we could provide.

I'm aware that this seems like a weird—even inappropriate—situation to relish. But that specific call brings back a cool morning with wet and clear early-fall light, a cup-of-coffee clarity. I wrote down the details and the man's phone number, then began to pick apart the problem like a geometric proof. The individual steps were complex, but I'd enjoyed story problems as a kid: make a list of each element in the situation and consider each section to tease apart the simplest solution.

"Legal issue re: benefits," I wrote. "Apply for waivers to hospital."

A few minutes later, Cathy arrived from a meeting, slamming the door behind her. She dropped her bags and furrowed her brow as she shuffled her phone messages. I asked her whether we knew anyone at the local legal aid office. She started to explain several different approaches and then stopped in midsentence. She stood with her mouth half open, thinking and looking at me as her inner third eye of policy simultaneously scanned a legislative loophole only she could see.

"This is really complicated," she said. "I'll meet with him; it will save time," she said. I reluctantly handed over the message pad. She checked her watch. "Let's talk about the organizing plan," she said.

The plan. I rooted around on my desk for my sketches. Fiction writing and politics overlapped here in the enjoyable, hypothetical bursts of motion onto the canvas of unsuspecting reality.

"I was thinking maybe we could hold a rally at whichever local hospital is worst in caring for the uninsured," I said, talking with my hands, sectioning off pieces of air to describe a multipart strategy. I could almost hear the pitched-yet-festive shouts of an imaginary demonstration echoing off the glass of a hospital foyer. "And we could do a bus tour of 'healthcare horrors' for local policy folks."

Cathy paused, half-smiling as she imagined the satisfying scene. Then a shadow of regret crossed her face, and the smile faded. "The hospitals really aren't the enemy," she said, watching me carefully. "We can't afford to damage our relationships with them."

That might have been the start of the sinking feeling in my gut, the free fall. How did one organize without a target, without a dragon to fight or an administrator to demonize? "What about holding a rally at the office of a local health insurance company?" I asked.

She sighed. Maybe she was frustrated at my need for a bad guy. "We don't monitor insurance. We monitor healthcare." In other words, we documented and drew attention to a lack, an absence. The only thing we could rage against was a void.

After a few weeks the immersion in the field of low-income healthcare had netted me a series of meetings. At most of these, I listened to concerns of Russian, Somali, and Latino immigrants from each of their social service agency advocates. We held roundtable meetings where we planned strategies for grant applications. I floundered as I took notes, realizing that as usual the grant opportunities were leading our work. Because there was funding available in the area of immigrant rights to healthcare, that became my de facto project, even though there were several people working on the effort already.

A woman named Ami came by the office one day to pick up some paperwork from Cathy to distribute to the Latino organization she worked for. She had golden brown ringlets of hair and blue eyes, and she clutched an enormous day planner.

Cathy did introductions, then said, "But you probably know each other already." We didn't, but Cathy's assumption was a safe one. In a midsized city like Columbus, the progressive organizers who stayed around for any length of time tended to know each other, regardless of the issue they worked on.

Ami and I sized each other up with shy eagerness. The number of women who stayed in organizing into their thirties was small, and they tended to fall into two camps. The first group, in my experience, struggled with burnout and big questions of their usefulness and politics and ethics on a daily basis. They wondered about how to get out or whether to get out, and asked themselves the same questions I was wondering, like can I sustain this? They had a sense of humor about their work, were searching like me for a healthy detachment and more of a full life than one consumed solely by politics. The members of the second group were martyrs to a particular organization, political orientation, or viewpoint and were in the process of being devoured by it. I was fighting hard to move from group two to group one.

"We should go out sometime," Ami said with a sincere smile. From the first coffee date, we discovered all the things we had in common, from family background to dilemmas with politics. Ami told me she wanted to introduce me to her friend Kathy, a mom with two young kids who'd just moved back into town to stay with her parents while she sorted out some issues with her husband. We started the slow process of friendship courting, revealing our stories and asking the other person for advice, then weighing the soundness of that advice to determine how much this person could be trusted.

One of my UHCAN tasks was to visit emergency rooms around the city to monitor their multilingual signage regarding the right to free care regardless of ability to pay. During my few months at UHCAN, I also compiled a report and planned a press conference; attended foundation meetings to pitch a healthcare project; wrote and submitted a grant to republish a brochure; networked with local immigration groups to collect information for a guide about immigrant healthcare for the local Somali, Russian, and Latino populations; organized meetings with local healthcare activists; visited several charity-care offices to collect applications and distributed them to people who needed them; and worked booths at local health fairs.

Strangely, my journal for early September 2000 records mostly single lines with the telltale stutter toward full stop: "UHCAN depression, lack of accomplishment."

It's hard to know whether UHCAN itself was the problem. Healthcare was kicking my ass in so many ways that I couldn't sort out the assaults. While others' hospital invoices covered my desk at work, I went home each night to confront myself as a case study of medical debt after a hospitalization that spring for a kidney infection.

One month into the UHCAN job, I wrote in my journal: "Sad about that hospital bill, I think. Makes me feel like I'll never get ahead." I think, as if even sadness wasn't mine to assert, as if my emotions were gooed and merged like taffy and I couldn't pull them apart.

One afternoon, I headed down the stairs and heaved open the church's heavy outer door. I paused to let a guy pass me on the steps. He was also leaving, carrying a Mac computer. He seemed a little sweaty, his eyes rolling a little in his head, but he smiled and nodded. Probably a repair guy. Shrug. I swallowed a twinge of awareness or suspicion in my gut. The sledgehammer of doom and depression said, "Fuck it. Just get out and go home." I held the door open for him. The next morning, the building erupted in shock because, of course, one of BREAD's new computers was missing.

What's clear from this distance is that I was approaching clinical depression of the repeat-offender variety. UHCAN needed the twenty-three-year-old version of me, not the pushing-thirty version who'd been worn down by every year since twenty-three. In late September I got a job offer at a local weekly newspaper, with benefits. I'd interviewed months earlier that summer and then hadn't heard anything and assumed the job was filled.

I gave Cathy my two weeks' notice, and I had to force myself to complete the simplest task. To make a list of projects for the next organizer, I had to grab a pen, haul my hand over to the legal pad, and not kill myself somewhere along the way. When Cathy left for meetings, I sat hunched over the yellow pages and called counselors to see if I could get an emergency counseling appointment.

"Do you have insurance?" they all asked.

"Self-pay," I replied.

September 23, 2000, was my last day at UHCAN. Before work I drove to St. Christopher's Catholic Church for a morning Mass. The priest intoned the Creed in a singsong from a thousand miles away. The blond-wood pews were empty except for me and three or four gray-headed men and women with sweaters and canes. My shoulders ached with knots of tension at the base of my neck. I used the blue and green stained glass windows, the smell of incense, and the waxlike statue of the Virgin Mary as last-ditch ploys to make myself breathe, to focus on something besides my own panic.

As happens so often with panic, I could see my emotions and the details of my life from far above, as if they were tiny, plastic, smiling people trapped in a snow globe. Trying to think myself out of a panic attack by imagining the rational response, *what I should be feeling right now*, is like trying to think myself from the outside to the inside of that snow globe. I knew I should be relieved to be done with UHCAN, happy to be starting another job. I drove to work.

Gold light, shaded by the yellowing leaves of a sycamore, streamed into the UHCAN office. Skate had been to the ER recently for a mystery ailment, a lump in his groin we thought might have been a hernia. It turned out to be a swollen gland. He left the ER hours later with a wave—no treatment needed, just a reminder to watch it. Now came more debt, and I had just started working on the charity-care application for him.

"It's kind of scary how much I use what I've learned here," I told Cathy. "But I wish he had insurance. I wish he'd see a doctor for all the stuff he complains about."

"Men will avoid healthcare at all costs," she said, laughing with eyes wide. "I can't even get my husband to see a doctor. He can be fainting or unable to hear in one ear, working surrounded by doctors in the ER, and he won't ask one of them to listen to his chest or give him a two-minute exam."

I couldn't fathom being part of healthcare and refusing that bounty. Bodies, germs, and dangers: to be alive was to be fucked, to be symptomatic meant prebankrupt. There was no way out; success meant you had to pay attention, pay attention, pay attention.

Four days later I sat in a psychiatric emergency room called Netcare. I studied the red-orange tiles of the floor, holding Skate's hand—I was past worrying whether he thought I was crazy. We waited for hours, watching a raving teenager on acid wrestle with his parents, waiting for my name to be called, knowing it would be okay.

The snow-globe feeling had a name here, and I said my panic in a familiar rosary as I sat in the Netcare clinician's office. I remember a large room like a lab or work area. There was a window; there was sunlight. I repeated the string of episodes that only made sense here: panic since age twenty, Zoloft since age twenty, depression since maybe age seven or eight, chronic with six or seven attempts to stop medication, six or seven relapses. It took maybe five minutes. They knew what they were seeing: a woman who, despite all evidence to the contrary, knew enough to recognize her own familiar emergencies and who was not scared by the furniture in that place. Admitting it was the only problem, and that was done. They could tell from my measured recitation that I was the easiest patient.

A woman or a man in a white paper coat handed me samples of Zoloft in a plain, white paper bag and—bless you, bless you—a small slip of paper bearing a prescription to tide me over until the insurance coverage kicked in at my new job. The small, plain, white bag was the size of a lunch bag, with a flat bottom so that it stood up by itself. It reminded me of everything good from childhood: candy, small toys, and unexpected happiness.

The next morning, I drove to my first day of work as a reporter. I stopped on the way to smoke a cigarette, another act like morning Mass, not a habit, just an attempt to adopt a new ritual of calm. I left the white paper bag of sample medications on the passenger seat, like a copilot, for comfort. That day, borrowing someone else's computer, I worked like a maniac, got a story assignment from an editor, and turned it around in three hours. My new boss gave me a look that said, "We don't really work that hard around here."

My mom arrived from Illinois that night to help scrape together her twenty-nine-year-old daughter, the woman beneath the master's degree who was still the same anxious kid. We rented Mansfield Park because I needed nothing of this century. We ate take-out chocolate cake with mocha icing. These are the things, remember, that are worth living for. Past caring whether I was pathetic, I was able to sleep, finally. I dreamt that political radicals denounced me for being counterrevolutionary because I was taking pills again.

Almost a decade later, a Web search reveals to me that UHCAN appears to have survived and thrived. Cathy is the executive director, and the new mission statement seems honed and focused, narrowed to issues of advocacy and creation of resources. The materials

I helped create are outdated and no longer available online. What I find of myself left in UHCAN's online memory is one statement in its chronology from the late 1990s: "As the prospects for real reform dimmed later in the decade, UHCAN helped keep the bells tolling for health care justice through its quarterly newsletter, national conferences, and relationship with state and local health care justice groups." The panic in my chest, the doom, and lack of direction that I took to be personal failings—maybe that's what it feels like when prospects dim.

I stopped by a florist to order a bouquet of yellow and white flowers for the staff at Netcare. The woman behind the counter listened to me and then wrote on the card, "Thank you for saving my life." She looked up and asked, "Do you want to sign it?" and I shook my head.

When I received my health insurance benefits packet from my new job, I held the nine-by-twelve-inch white envelope close to my chest, not realizing my benefits wouldn't kick in for another few months. At home I thumbed through the certificate of benefits to find the number for Magellan, the coordinator for my mental health benefits, and called them with a nervous thrill as though I were asking for a first date.

They couldn't find me in the system, of course, because it was too soon. I wanted to leap headfirst into my new relationship. An operator put me on hold, and I hummed to a Muzak version of a jangling song I recognized from high school. It was comforting and familiar. I nodded my head vaguely.

"Hey now, hey now . . ." I sang to myself. Oh, it was Crowded House, the New Zealanders. I used to have this tape. It must be a good sign. Then Finn sang, "Don't dream it's over," and my chest seized. No, it's not over. Why would you say it's "over"? Over.

Breathe.

I quickly learned that I was not a natural at the house style of the weekly paper, which was sort of snarky and apolitical, funny and deadpan. At our weekly story meetings, I pitched nerdy, complicated ideas about regional planning and environmentalism and healthcare, most of which were thoroughly rewritten before appearing in print. My most lauded story of that year would detail a lawsuit filed by a local woman whose Victoria's Secret thigh-high tights stuck to her sweaty legs and peeled off strips of skin when removed.

On the upside, I met the arts editor, Jenny, who was cooler than cool and had dyed black hair. She was a drummer in a local band and had a sharp eye with text. She dropped by my cubicle to compliment me on a story I wrote or a dress I bought at a garage sale. Our coffees and movie dates began to resemble life organizational-and-planning meetings, where we reviewed dreams, goals, and agendas. She was newly married, and I had just moved into a drafty half of a duplex with Skate. Jenny and I talked domestic negotiations and relationships as we both pulled away from the club scene and the bar scene and toward writing and art, nudging ourselves into some alternate version of adulthood that might make us feel calmer and happier.

Using the blind instrument of my own happiness and sanity as a rough yardstick, the weekly paper job rated low, even shellacked in a regular coating of Zoloft and augmented by the huge carrot of benefits. Each week was an escalating pitch of panic to accumulate story ideas, chase sources, and crank out stories. The pounding of the keyboard nine to five each day killed my desire to write anything of my own. It felt like phantom limb syndrome, an ache over something that wasn't there. Even before I'd settled into my health insurance provider network by around December, I had submitted an application to the MFA program in creative writing at Ohio State University.

"I know I shouldn't do this, but I can't stop myself," I said to Jenny one afternoon as she drove us toward the movie theater in the early winter of 2001. We were talking about the MFA program; I'd just gotten my acceptance. I wanted it like a drug, but jumping ship from a good, stable job with benefits and career potential was exactly the opposite of the previous plan.

At a stoplight, she put out her cigarette, rolled up the window, and looked at me with her ice blue eyes. "And your gut tells you . . . ?"

PRESCRIPTIONS

We fled from campus to someone's living room and sat around the glowing porthole of CNN, peering into New York's ashy hell. In a somber toast to our new lives in wartime, someone brought out the pot, rolled a joint. I drank my ice water and passed the joint without inhaling, knowing pot would make me still more anxious and unsettled.

I numbly wandered into our host's bathroom. On a low wire rack piled with bath products beneath the sink, I spotted an amber bottle of prescription-strength allergy medication. I picked up the bottle of Claritin. Like a cache of powerful larvae, the ovals nestled densely. In a flash of denial and prosaic problem-solving mania, I numbly multitasked, stole, and became overly involved with Skate's uninsured sinuses. I opened the bottle and fished out one pill with the tip of a moistened finger. I put the pill in my pocket.

On the back porch, women's palms exuded muffled clacks as cell phones clicked shut like muted castanets. Calls to New York, where husbands and lovers worked and lived, could not be completed as dialed. Our arms twined around our torsos as if to hold in our organs. We chewed on our moisturized cuticles with the edges of our white teeth, and our eyes scanned the still and flawless sky. Someone changed the channel to Matt Lauer and Katie Couric, who sat at a round table strewn with papers and gripped bottles of spring water.

Comfort looked like those plastic bottles of water, like a plastic bottle filled with prescription medication. Comfort to my friends looked like ice cubes glinting in glasses, like the lava-red glowing tip of burning marijuana. Comfort looked like things we could put in our mouths to solve the small problems.

A strictly economist view of restitution might grant me absolution if I were to find that almost stranger, who was then a graduate teaching assistant in training like me, and pay her for one Claritin. The allergy pill was available only by prescription back in 2001. She probably shelled out a co-pay of $15 for thirty pills, so I might get off easy with a bill of fifty cents. Claritin can now be purchased over the counter for about $1 a pill. Either way, the financial damage I inflicted on this woman was minimal, and I hasten to add that I didn't even take a hit off her joint, which would have cost more than fifty cents per toke. But wait, the pot was offered freely in a ritual of panic and bonding. Sadly, nobody hands out antihistamines as hors d'oeuvres. So the meaning of my action contains the crime: I took something that wasn't given in order to give something that wasn't requested.

I might claim my intervention was motivated by love and concern. But I could not have been more selfish. Skate sniffled daily, red-eyed while holding power tools, working outside in hay fever season. That morning, he had been up on scaffolding under the bright blue sky repairing a chimney when the towers collapsed. The house was in a rough neighborhood; when a crack addict wandered by and screamed, "Man, they're bombing New York!" he thought it a crack fantasy and shook his head.

How is it possible, in a state of national emergency, to steal an allergy pill?

Skate and I had gotten engaged three months earlier in midsummer 2001. I started a wedding to-do list in a spiral notebook. I collected prices, added up figures, and then shaved them down to bring the total in under $4,000. Jenny gave me the name of the woman who'd baked her wedding cake and shared her tips on photographers and caterers, each with price quotes that made me laugh out loud.

Skate had started his own carpentry business, and the jobs were slow coming in. I had realized that my job as a graduate teaching assistant at Ohio State would bring in less than $1,000 a month. Every wedding option required a cheaper, duct-taped version: centerpieces morphed into mason jars holding Dollar Store votive candles, and tablecloths appeared one by one from garage sales.

I carried the wedding binder with me and ticked off tasks between meetings for Jobs with Justice, the community-labor coalition I'd helped to start. I piloted my car from one union hall to another. If I had a pocket of ten free minutes, I would make a call to a source for a freelance magazine article I was working on.

In our living room one evening, I packed my bag for a labor meeting, glancing at the clock as I shoved the wedding binder in with my labor folders. Through my Jobs with Justice work, I'd received a paid contract to do some community organizing on a campaign to unionize Wal-Mart, and I was headed out to talk with religious leaders about their role in an upcoming rally.

Skate looked up from the television. "You're leaving again?"

I probably said something like, "It's just this week that's busy. Next week is wide open." But I would go nonetheless, feeling guilty for my perverse urges toward labor unionization and writing, my need for faces and people and effort and meetings.

American flags blanketed the facades of buildings on the main roads leading to campus that fall. A group of women met outside near a main campus intersection every Friday afternoon to hold signs to protest the drive to war. We modeled ourselves on a group of Israeli women who protested their country's actions against Palestine and stood for an hour in silence.

I held my poster-board sign that read, "Stop the War," and watched the insides of my head roll like ocean swells. The traffic clogged in rippling rows of brake lights at red lights and rushed forward at each green. I mulled over the tugs and pulls and to-do lists eating at my day. How could I explain to Skate, much less to myself, that a rally or a picket line gave me a sense of a foundation? At least in those hours, I knew that we were doing something, that I was among people who would act.

I looked down at my left hand curled around the poster board. The white-gold engagement ring on my finger felt heavy and serious. Skate had given me a diamond from his grandmother. I'd paid for the wedding band myself, in our typical fashion—cash strapped and catch-as-catch-can. But no one needed to know that. Professors and graduate students and labor union presidents could all look at it and see, I imagined, the hand of an adult, not a girl, not the scraggly waif I sometimes saw myself as, not the scraping-by activist. Strange that I would rebel so often and then hunger for the legitimacy and safety of these symbols, thinking that the symbols themselves meant my life would change.

One evening that fall, the congestion from Skate's head settled into his lungs and then into what sounded like bronchitis. Without insurance, allergy pills required a $60 office visit and another $50 or so for a prescription. I may have brought him tea or cough drops, but beneath a look of sympathy was a fester of calculation. I waited, watching his face, for a calm and open minute in which he might listen to me.

"You know," I said, "there are the public clinics, where we could get you in to see someone. It's sliding scale. Then at least you'd have a prescription, maybe some samples." I knew with an almost painful clarity about the range of options for low-cost healthcare available in the city. I also knew that, with a quick income verification form, we could write to the manufacturer of the allergy pill and get Skate on a regular free shipment. I had to hold myself back from laying out the full battle plan.

Skate shook his head. He was used to the sickness, and the time required for waiting, calls, visits, and forms would drive him crazy. The last thing he wanted was to be sitting somewhere in an uncomfortable waiting room chair when he could be working, skating, painting, living his life.

As a self-employed carpenter, Skate worked on ladders and leaned over shrieking table saws. He saved money by treating a minor medical problem as a carpentry challenge. When he smashed his thumb with a hammer, the swelling made his thumb unusable and pickle sized. So he took a tiny drill bit and drilled through the thumbnail down into his finger. Pus and blood shot out of the hole in an orange gush. He explained that this had happened before and that the thumbnail usually turned black and fell off after one of these procedures. He kept a collection of pierced and blackened thumbnails in a film canister.

He didn't need insurance. It was a waste of money, he said. By even mentioning the need for insurance and its cousin, tragedy, he felt I'd woken the evil sleeping voodoo genie of death. I tried to keep quiet, to wait for the universe to deliver a solution, while I envisioned his circular saw slipping, creating horrible, maiming visions, slippery with his uninsured blood.

"You can add me to your policy after we get married," he said.

I shook my head. I'd already considered this. The wedding wasn't until fall of the next year, and even then it would be too expensive. So I tried to offer solutions. I ordered pamphlets and price quotes for catastrophic health insurance policies. I probably left them strategically placed on the kitchen table for him to look at.

Insurance once carried the double meaning of "betrothal, troth-plighting, engagement to marry." Four hundred years after those first British policies protected from the losses of shipwreck and fire, engagement and insurance were still synonymous, so much so that insurance dilemmas shaped every major life decision: when to get married and why, when to leave, how to leave, when to have children and with whom. I knew marriage offered no ironclad shelter from the storms and catastrophes of life, but the promise of being united by an insurance plan gave marriage an additional sheen of solidity. Facing the health gods as a team seemed to increase our odds of survival as prey.

Skate and I had different definitions of safety and different needs for security, but I assumed in this case I was being a neurotic worrier. I didn't define this gap between us as a difference in values that might have told me something about our relationship. Instead, I saw it as a practical problem. After fretting and stewing, I pulled out the biggest gun I had: I told him I would not marry him unless he had insurance. I knew I was going to marry him anyway, but it forced him to sign up for a catastrophic-illness plan with a $2,000 deductible. When he got the policy, I paid half of the premium each month, in recognition of the fact that the policy protected my mental health more than it guarded his physical well-being.

We sat in the dark wooden pews at the back of the dimly lit church, listening to Cathy run down the schedule for the press conference. We—the group of UHCAN volunteers and healthcare advocates—would occupy the street corners near the statehouse to explain the bill coming up that would widen access to affordable healthcare for uninsured adults. I was still in regular contact with Cathy and on her volunteer roster.

Cathy's new UHCAN organizer handed me a megaphone. "Just be loud," she said, and I nodded. The organizer moved through the pews, handing out bandages splotched with fake blood. A few kids near the back entryway stuck Band-Aids all over their T-shirts and arms.

I stopped to chat with an older man I knew from UHCAN coalition work who leaned back in a pew with his eyes closed, hand gently resting on the curve of his cane. He'd had to declare bankruptcy due to medical bills. He was great to have in the UHCAN activist pool as someone who'd seen the effects of the current system firsthand.

"Remember to act sick, Malcolm!" I said with a smile.

He opened his eyes and looked at me. "I am sick," he said quietly.

I mumbled some apology and marshaled my troupe of volunteers out of the church. But Malcolm's quiet reminder cut a layer of humbled sadness through that day, made me remember how often as an organizer I had condensed people's pain into talking points, how necessary and yet how ridiculous it was to use humans as case studies to make rhetorical points.

Maybe my blindness came about because I looked only beyond myself for proof of the problems I wanted to fight. With all my energy directed outward—toward the steel workers in Marion, Ohio, who were getting injured on the job and losing fingers or toward the popcorn-factory workers getting lung infections from inhaling clouds of powdered butter—I suppose it was easy to see my problems as minimal. That separation between me and the people who were truly in trouble helped to fuel my early activism, my shock at the extreme cases, the tragedies I could not imagine living through, the stories we used to silence the crowd and the reporters at press conferences. I was not one of those people. I was pretty healthy, getting by, privileged to have access to healthcare. All I wanted was to spread the wealth.

Each morning in that first year of graduate school, I swallowed a little red pill with my coffee, an over-the-counter Sudafed decongestant. Extra pills rolled around in the corners of my purse, like little red-hot candies, collecting lint.

I bought a box of decongestants during each trip to the grocery store. I laughed when I saw the pharmacist pause before handing me Sudafed to check his list of suspicious customers.

"No," I said, "I don't run a meth lab. I'm really just that stuffed up." Unless I cleared my sinuses, my head would feel like a casserole, and I couldn't concentrate on my reading or my writing but could count on sinus infections and days of lost productivity.

I visited a doctor at the campus health center and described the symptoms of obvious seasonal allergies: the runny nose, scratchy throat and ears, buzzing head. The doctor sat diagonally to my right behind a desk. He nodded, stroked his chin, and flipped through my chart.

"Hmmm," he said. "I don't see any history of allergies in your chart."

"Correct. I've never received treatment for allergies. Because I'm lying," I might have said to the doctor. "Because this is not for me. Because life is not going the way I'd planned. Because the game is not going in my favor, and so I'm going to cheat."

The doctor shrugged and wrote me a prescription for allergy pills. "I hope this helps," he said.

I held my purposeful little grad-student shoulder bag, filled with pens and appointments and shopping lists. I sat in the doctor's office and reached for my prescription, which meant one thing: a vial of pills I could take home to Skate.

I stepped down the stairs toward the brick path, moving slowly and carefully to contain my joy. I was in like an undetected thief. I paid—a song, a nothing—and stuffed the amber bottle wrapped in its white paper baggie and assorted warning labels and receipts into my tote bag, flooded with a sense of relief, wealth, and well-being. I wanted to dash home and hand the vial over like a prize. I possessed the ability to change and master the symptoms of illness, the illusion or reality of helping to heal.

Children steal because they want to even the equation; they often can't imagine that one day in the natural course of time, they will grow into power. When I was small, I stole penny candy and plastic grapes from fruit arrangements in the upstairs arts-and-crafts section of Bruns' drugstore. I squeezed a plastic purple bulb, held the open hole against my skin, and then let go. Suction adhered the grape-bulb tightly to my arm or forehead like a boil or a massive wart. The small objects of my theft represented my secret will. They held mysterious significance, and I wanted them in order to see myself.

As I got older, the infrequent targets of my theft became more symbolic. I took an expensive name-brand shirt from a friend during a sleepover because I lusted not so much for the shirt (which was unattractive and of the Coca-Cola brand strangely popular in the Midwest in the late eighties) as for the elusive status it seemed to promise. I mailed the shirt back to her later with a gift and an apology. But the damage was done and she never replied. In my twenties I was an infrequent shoplifter, hitting the jewelry racks at the Dollar Store and Urban Outfitters when my life seemed particularly bleak and unadorned.

I applied to well-paying corporate jobs and found myself unworthy and unqualified. I worried that maybe I had never been middle-class enough and did not know it, or maybe I had squandered my chance. As a temporary receptionist, I wore a sacklike black skirt I bought for a dollar from Goodwill. I did not mind Goodwill or even taking things from the trash and the curb when they appealed to me and fit; that was fun. But most of the small thefts were things I did not desperately need. My low income created a general fog of lack that made anything with a price tag into a promise of forbidden comfort.

I stole markers from my job in Boston at the photo-processing store. I stole soap and shampoo from the youth home. I stole stacks of Post-it notes from office jobs, pens from doctors' offices, and a vinyl drink coaster from an expansive conference room table at a pointless job interview in Chicago. I liberated things from the Man. Or else maybe I wanted to be the Man. I resented people who had disposable income. I wanted pretty things, and the world owed me these treats, which it dangled just beyond the clear barriers of department store windows.

I lusted after safety, but I also hated those who had what I wanted. At the same time, I hated those who had set up these barriers and tests, making life so hard. I can't tell now which of these emotions was stronger. Even though I am safe today, I can close my eyes and feel a stripe of residual orange anger down the center of my belly.

And here is the truth another way: I stole that first Claritin from bitterness, and lied to get the bottle from joy. I stole the first pill because it was an easy mark, not because it would actually improve my situation. That first theft was motivated by spite, as if I'd run a car key along the shiny surface of a Mercedes, because it represented the other life I wanted for myself and my fiancé, the life in which we were both insured and enfolded in that sense of tangible and bodily security I craved. I took it also because I was angry he didn't seem to want that life. I was frustrated and impatient and enraged at the world for failing to conform to my image of how things should be. I took it because I was afraid we would never get there. I took it because I was angry with myself for being tempted, because I felt too old to be scrounging for pills.

The whole bottle—that was joy, a victimless crime. Faking a prescription is an offense that carries a sentence of up to a $5,000 fine and five years in jail. Most people create fake prescriptions to feed their addictions to controlled substances. People who fake ailments to get narcotics are addicts who need help, or they are criminals taking advantage of other people's addictions.

I was high on my own thrifty resourcefulness, my ability to take care of a problem with the dormant power of my student health insurance card. I wanted to help. But more than anything else, I wanted the worry to stop, so much so that I was willing to easily slide from misdemeanor to felony. I then stuffed the crime as far as possible under my layers of to-do lists, until I could barely feel that one Claritin, just as the princess felt the pea.

Seven years later, an allergist would finally tell me that a decade of Sudafed could have damaged my heart. My first good benefits package and safe job—years in the future—would prompt me to investigate all those nagging minor problems of my own body. This could only occur after medicine became less of a battlefield and I stopped stepping into a doctor's office with dukes up and guns drawn, waiting to get hammered with a bill.

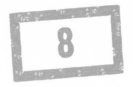

8

EMPLOYEE + CHILD(REN)

If you don't have the money to support a kid, don't have one. Those words must have floated from my twenty-something mouth between sips of beer at some bar. In this nonsensical model of sex and procreation, true foreplay would begin with the slow accumulation of quarters and dollars. At a certain dollar amount, the red flashing lights of this pinball game would swirl, and the egg would rocket around a Plexiglas turbo-track fallopian tube on the way to the extra bonus round.

Give this pinball wizard two more beers and she'd admit the truth in a woozy whisper: "I can't imagine how anyone saves enough money to have a kid. How do people do it? Please, God and Tinker Bell, sprinkle some pixie dust over here and, like, let the answer reveal itself."

I passed thirty and this magic wad of baby cash had mysteriously failed to accumulate. The exact price tag of "enough to have a baby" was revealed neither in the *Girl Scout Handbook* nor in Sleater-Kinney lyrics, although newspaper articles made me scoff at a figure of around $100,000 per child. In 2001 I made a list of my own options, contemplating present and future earning potential, months and years of fertility in a kind of story problem:

(1) A thirty-two-year-old woman's take-home pay is about $986 a month. If her husband is a thirty-three-year-old, self-employed

carpenter, he takes home about $900 a month after paying for his own benefits. Is this enough money for a baby?

(2) Add the issue of maternity leave: If this woman waits to reproduce, she will start a job at age thirty-three; pregnancy and employer ire would begin at age thirty-four, at which time she would receive at most six weeks' unpaid leave. If she gets pregnant in graduate school at age thirty-two, the woman would receive no paid leave but could flex her schedule enough to stay home (unpaid leave plus adjunct teaching and part-time proofreading) for six months.

(3) Take into account the fact that this woman's biological window of safest and healthiest reproductive capacity would close at age thirty-five. Should she gamble, instead, that a solution would reveal itself before the end of that window?

"We're thrifty people," said Skate. "We'll figure it out."

We *were* thrifty people, and we managed to greet the wedding guests in the fall of 2001 at a public rose garden with a wedding that cost under $3,000, including dress and rings.

Brooke, my friend from the student nonprofit, flew out from New York the day before the wedding, making her first trip to the Midwest for me. She met me at our apartment with eyes wide. "This place isn't so bad," she said in shock. "I think I saw some lesbians." Monica came in with coffee and scones from the corner coffee shop, and I sent her off with my sister Nicole to make a trip to the rented reception hall with decorations and paper plates. Later, as I messed up and redid my nail polish, Monica and Brooke chatted about law school and the work they hoped to do as public defenders. Sharad barreled in after an all-night drive from a day of work in Boston, sat through the ceremony, gave me a bear hug, and then had to get in the car and leave for another job.

The day before, I had sent out an e-mail labor update and had been chastened by a labor activist for not immersing myself in my wedding. I'd cleared away a few days for a honeymoon in southeast Ohio and had a full to-do list stocked for my return. To me, my work and my wedding weren't separate activities; my organizing skills had made the wedding possible.

After the ceremony, we had a quick meal of barbeque and mac'n' cheese donated by Joe, a friend who was a cook at a local restaurant. We cleared up the paper plates and then went home to our garage, where the only reception I wanted was a really good party. We set up the folding tables, opened the garage door, and put mozzarella cheese sticks in the oven. We plugged in the white Christmas lights we'd thrown over the trellis Skate made, and I kicked off my shoes. The grass was wet from the rain we'd had for days, but the night was clear and cool. Skate made a fire in the backyard, and Nicole helped me light candles and set them in paper bags to line our front walk.

A few Jobs with Justice activists stopped by to offer hugs and presents. Jenny brought her husband to say hello and have a beer. Skate's friends launched fireworks and presented him with a $600 saw they'd all chipped in to buy. Kathy and Ami sat together near the fire, laughing at a joke told by Skate's best friend. Barefoot on the lawn, I drank from a bottle of cheap champagne. What warmed me that night was not primarily a notion of romantic coupledom. Instead, I remember hugging my sister and my brother, being glad that Nicole could meet Kathy and Ami and Jenny, that a group of people had pulled together and helped us make a wedding.

I had one big thing going for me, a prize even more glittery and valuable than financial stability: health insurance. I sported a gang consciousness about my university-sponsored insurance card, and I would have gladly purchased a satin jacket in our colors with my name embroidered on the breast ("administered by Klais Benefits" and, later, "MEGA Benefits" or something like that). Other people got worked up about Ohio State football, but I felt more nationalistic and rabidly emotional about my status as a health insurance "have" in the world of "have-nots." This, I realize, seems to contradict the "Healthcare for All" bumper sticker on my car—but really, both stem from the same source. I still rabidly want everyone to have healthcare. But while we were waiting for the insurance rapture, I quietly reveled in the knowledge that my own gallbladder might explode and someone would be required to fix it.

Like the drama of Ohio State football and its shifting wins and tragic defeats, my healthcare nationalism was whipped up like a rousing postgame riot precisely by those moments in which healthcare dashed my wildest hopes. Somehow that undertone of fear, like worrying about whether the quarterback might have a bad morning or blow out his elbow, made me cling with fonder devotion to the plastic rectangle in my wallet.

Imagine my ecstasy when I flipped through my certificate of benefits toward the "M" section, seeking "Maternity." My vision became spotted with fireworks of blue and purple as I forgot to breathe . . . oh dear God, please let this be good . . . It's GOOD! The ref raised his hands, the kick shot between the goal posts, and I got to have a baby for the grand total of $300. I responded silently to my earlier social-policy pronouncements: *Yep, I can afford to have a baby. In fact, I have money left over.*

That winter, Skate and I bought a house. In other words, a creative mortgage broker gave a graduate student, who had good credit and was making $18,000 a year, a loan for a $70,000 fixer-upper. Our neighbors divided themselves evenly between the stuck and the crack addicted. I had this idea in my head, unarticulated but moving me like a tectonic plate, that home ownership was the other precursor to having a child. Never mind the fact that we moved from a safe university neighborhood to one where gunfire could be heard every night, where we watched the rentals cycle between merely shambling and boarded up. Somehow, debt against a collapsing piece of property meant adulthood. Maybe it was the Catholic in me that yearned to follow some of the rules in hopes that a sense of security would await on the other side.

I tried for a nanosecond to get pregnant in the spring of 2002 and then got exhausted and dispirited by school deadlines and writing and winter. Stress or worry apparently led to the mother of all sinus infections, a throbbing swamp head of nonproductivity. It was early March in Ohio, and I could barely haul myself onto the bus to go to the health center. We tried regular antibiotics and moved quickly up to a ridiculous blast of toxicity emblazoned with a sticker that read, "Do Not Take If Pregnant." The doctor asked if there was any chance I could be pregnant. "No way," I said. "No baby could live through this."

I started the pills, and after a few days I kept finding myself staring at the grid of the calendar as if I was forgetting to do something. I called my friend Kathy. "How did you feel when you were pregnant?" I asked.

"The first time, I felt fine. The second time, I felt like a truck had hit me," she said. She paused. "Sinuses tend to react to pregnancy, along with everything else. Do you think you might need more information about this?" I love it when Kathy switches over into her counselor-job voice, because that's when I can tell I am being clinically stupid.

"I know, I know," I said. "I'll go get a test."

I peed on the plastic stick, saw a plus sign for positive, and set it down carefully on the edge of the bathroom sink. I got up with a strange numbness and went back to my office to work on an article that was due in a few hours. Once the sentences were looped and knit together, once the article was proofread and e-mailed off to my editor, then I would sit back and assess.

My first three months of pregnancy left me with a close-up memory of our brown couch, its scratchy woven surface flecked with a subtle rainbow of colored threads in the tan family. I began to have a new appreciation for this palette of blues, oranges, and greens with my face pressed right up to it for hours at a time. Every once in a while I stood up and shuffled into the kitchen to shove saltines into my mouth.

At month four I lay in bed and felt the ocean of nausea wane. Finally, I could think. The morning sunlight dappled the bedspread. Wow, I'm going to be a mom. What would it be like to have a teenager of my very own to tell me to fuck off? What would it be like to deal with school registration, all the daily logistics . . . ? My windpipe tightened and adrenaline surged as my heart contracted in red fury, as if my peripheral vision had spotted a vulture circling or my hearing registered the rumble of a semitruck about to burst into our living room. I sat up. Wait. . . . Oh, shit. Another human body heading out into the world meant that I had to find another health insurance card.

I called Human Resources at the university and discovered, as I'd expected, that there were no maternity benefits for graduate students. I researched the issue and found a few unionized campuses where the idea was being floated, but that demand was still years in the future in the United States. While my cousin in Germany had a year of maternity benefits paid by the state, my employer on campus looked at my due date and then crossed off two weeks after that at the end of the semester. She told me that if I missed work due to the birth of my child, I would have to make up the time after he was born.

The summer morphed into a bump in my lap, and I could finally tell people why I'd been acting so weird. I started doing that pregnant-woman thing of rubbing my belly constantly, maybe because the stretched-tight skin itched. At labor coalition meetings or at rallies, some of the older union guys who had looked through me because they assumed I was some well-meaning nineteen-year-old suddenly stepped out of my way, held the door, got me a chair. I collected baby clothes at garage sales and pushed away the building sense that this mothering thing was going to take a huge chunk of time out of my mobility and my schedule.

In the summer of 2002 our labor coalition was finally certified as an official chapter by the national organization. We held an annual retreat for our leaders and board, and I was bitten by a sense of breathless impatience in these meetings. Standing in front of the flip chart with a permanent marker in my hand, I wanted to urge the coalition members to get to the point, to stop being so relaxed and chatting about their weekends. Time was running short, and my due date loomed as the day on which my life would spin out of control.

I usually save the entire nine-by-twelve-inch envelope of brochures and guides sent by each health insurance plan, because I worry that if I throw away the hospice brochure or the free bookmark, I might rattle the health insurance gods and attract the evil eye of benefits denial. Similarly, I have a hard time throwing away health brochures and certificates of coverage from the job before the job before the job before this one. I save them in a file and promise myself I will get around to sorting my mementos of coverage past.

In the almost-pristine package for my OSU policy documents, I easily located the excellent color-coded health insurance brochure, which was printed on substantial cardstock and finished with a half-gloss, half-matte surface that seemed to promise clinical efficiency administered with a human touch. Each column contained a benefits plan along with the total cost. The menu of options comforted me. My eyes glazed as I resisted reading the words on the benefits brochure. I held on to my fantasy of affordable coverage. Finally, anxiety tipped the balance and I focused on the text, printed in white seven-point font on a multicolored background.

The columns were headed with plan names like "Buckeye," "Ultimate," and "Choice Select." My eyes suddenly hurt, and I had to fight the urge to lie down on my soft, lovely bed. Why couldn't they come up with clearer plan names, like "Have the Butler Make This Decision," "Middle Eastern Student Who Will Be Deported before Seeing a Specialist," and "Horrifically Diseased and Forced to Pay Anything to Stay Alive"?

The chart's bottom row offered a string of numbers: the total cost for each color-coded plan. I avoided those figures and tried to decipher the bread-crumb trail of co-pays and deductibles to locate the thriftiest plan. There it was: "Buckeye Plus." I rewarded myself with a break for contemplation, then made a list of what I had to be grateful for: fresh bread, flowers, friends, and a baby on the way. Okay, I was spiritually prepared for a punch in the teeth. I dove back into the row titled "Employee + spouse + child(ren)" on the Buckeye Plus. I used my finger to trace the row across to the monthly employee cost: $893.00. My lungs and stomach hurled against each other in shock as if I'd plummeted down a roller-coaster track, and my son reacted on a five-second delay to the adrenaline surge in my bloodstream by aiming a strong kick to my thorax.

What would it feel like to work essentially without payment in exchange for healthcare? For a moment I was perversely tempted. Maybe it would be kind of purifying and monastic, a simple life in which I wouldn't be troubled with thoughts about extraneous luxuries like tampons or soap. Spending that much was so ridiculous it was almost a pleasure to contemplate, a binge purchase on something I coveted.

I mentally tossed my husband overboard and moved to the next "Buckeye" option, "Employee + child(ren)." This amount was more reasonable: it would allow me to pay my half of the rent, and I'd have an extra $30 left over for lottery tickets, malt liquor, and cyanide.

The ultrasound heartbeat thrummed like an ocean explorer's submarine engine. The technician clicked his mouse on dark circles on the screen, marking eyes, hands, and feet. Each checkup and squirt of bluish goo on my widening belly seemed to present a small expansion of an unoccupied zone, a land of safety I had not imagined, motivated only by itself.

Nobody told me it was okay to grow a baby. I just went and did it—the ultimate do-it-yourself project. Inside there in gray splotches, I saw the narrow, pointed chin and wide eyes I would always recognize as the marks of my son's face. Most of the time, I couldn't even bring myself to contemplate him—a person—being in there. A boy. I told myself I would believe it was a real baby when I saw a real baby. But he kicked with impressive firepower, rolled like thunder, banged into my ribs, as if he knew he needed to shake me up to get my attention and derail my to-do lists.

In my various battles on my own behalf, I had focused often on the odds of failure, on the possible reasons why someone would refuse my demands, why the phone call might not be returned, the article might be rejected, or the coalition meeting might go awry. I had focused on finding loopholes and slipping into security undetected.

But a baby is an excellent coalition partner. It takes what it needs and asks for more. Its strength is in its need. It yells louder than anyone else and demands attention. It never apologizes or feels guilty for its need. It models boldness. I saw it feeding off of me from the inside, busting out the walls of myself to make room. That blatant taking inspired me. The weight resting on my hips forced me to widen my stance.

One night that summer, I rang the doorbell to Kathy's parents' house. Kathy appeared at the screen door, then hugged me and beamed, looking down at my belly. "You look great," she said. "And I have clothes for you."

She lugged a blue plastic storage bin out onto the screened-in back porch, and we sat down. Gnats pinged their bodies into the glowing lightbulb above us, and she lifted out stack after stack of folded maternity clothes. Each one came with a story, most of them being passed from sisters-in-law through neighbors and friends in Minnesota to California to Ohio, to sisters, then to friends, and back. I balked at the jeans with the huge elasticized panels in the front, and she said, "Just you wait. It looks insane, but soon you won't be able to fit into anything else."

Deeper and deeper into the bin, it became clear we were excavating decades of pregnancies. The bottom layer was a riot of garish faux-plaid patterns printed on silk, all adorned with huge plastic gold buttons and shoulder pads. "Whoa, that's the eighties down there," I said. "I'll pass on those."

We laid out stacks of the clothes we thought would fit me. Kathy laid a hand on the cotton of a summer dress. "I remember wearing this when I was five months pregnant," she said. "We were moving from Chicago up to Minnesota, and neither of us had insurance. I had no idea what we were going to do. I threw out my back from the tension of the eight-hour drive."

I could almost see the bugs splattered on the windshield of that northward trek, and I imagined the undercurrent of tension that must have run between Kathy and her then-husband. It was unavoidable, the scary pressure of bringing a new human into the world, knowing you didn't quite have the bases covered. You kept looking into each other's eyes for extra reassurance, knowing all the while you wouldn't find it there, the anxiety reflecting and amplifying like light beams bouncing between mirrors.

I started to cry for either the first or seventh time that day. I pressed the heels of my hands into the corners of my eyes. "God," I said. "I know. I don't know what . . ." And I trailed off, because the questions were so big I couldn't even finish the sentence. Maybe it was the baby pressing on my esophagus, causing heartburn and a choking feeling, as if I were a toothpaste tube being squeezed from the bottom up.

That summer, I attended mother-to-be classes on breast-feeding and baby care. I shyly looked around the rooms of women for a sign of something familiar besides a rounded belly. When I saw the hint of a tattoo peeking out from under a shirt sleeve, the snug pull of a thrift-store vintage T-shirt, the worn fabric of a unisex messenger bag, or the ripple of beaded necklaces and silver chains, I would waddle over and say hi.

As I stood on the edge of a small knot of these alternative women, hands resting on bellies, the conversation dipped into the questions that faced them: whether to give birth at home, how to make organic baby food, whether to immunize, whether or not to go back to work after the baby arrived, or whether to ever work again.

I nodded but kept silent on those questions. I had no time to puree organic sweet potatoes, no money for a home-delivery service for cloth diapers.

"What does your partner or husband do?" I would ask.

The responses—"He's in sales" or "He's an engineer"—often came with a half smile and a half-bashful glance, as if to say, "I can't believe I got all normal." I never met the husbands, those punks who cleaned up real nice, the degreed band boys with a knack for cubicle life.

Some of these women forwarded me e-mail newsletters about the dangers of immunization, about composing a birth plan that specified minimal medical intervention. They wanted to keep medicine at arm's length, and I wanted into its embrace.

Like planning an illegal escape across no-man's-land to the border of another country, my husband, baby, and I would have to go separately into the land of healthcare security. I would toss my baby in a basket through one hole, clamber up through a niche, and hope

I could find my husband on the other side. We were legally a family. But in the most practical measure—the question of which safety net sheltered our physical bodies, which route would bring us to safety—we were a failed family already, a split and fractured group making its way across the border with cards in different fonts and colored logos, sent from different addresses, with different procedures and co-pays.

The signs were obvious: I was low-income, with a low-income spouse. I was a sleeping-beauty welfare queen just waiting to flutter open her long lashes and claim her vast royal holdings. But I could not be needy, for I wore the mantel of ultimate privilege. I toiled in the land of the book. I taught students at a university, the lordly and noble profession grouped around green courtyards and within fortress-shaped buildings. I played a central role in passing on culture and knowledge to the next generation.

I cherished a view of myself as purely progressive, but I couldn't imagine that my name would fit on an application for Temporary Assistance to Needy Families or for the Women, Infants, and Children nutritional program. I could fix this, I reasoned. All I needed was a little bit of research.

The pile of healthcare quotes on my desk grew. Each brochure was emblazoned with cursive slogans like "We Want to Help" and "Your Final Healthcare Solution" (I'm not kidding—that one was real), over stock photos of smiling doctors and ethnically diverse, freakishly happy patients.

The plan options inside these folders, however, were low budget, printed in plain black type on thin white paper, not a pleasure to examine. The rows and columns offered fewer choices, each of which asked me to wager whether my kid was *really* going to fall down the stairs or get hit by a car, or whether I was just being a worrywart about this whole frailty-of-flesh-and-blood thing. I thought my husband's individual plan might give us some kind of break for being long-term customers. The benefits administrator, whom I'll call Kelly and whom I really was on a first-name basis with, suggested the $2,000-deductible policy. Deductible is such a great word, like describing a human being as "die-able."

"Thanks, Kelly," I said. "I'll think about it." And I did. I brooded. I worried and added figures and subtracted our monthly bills and mortgage, and I saw that there was no well-baby program for the individual policies and that I would essentially be paying for everything out of pocket anyway. It was cheaper to not have insurance at all, and yet I would have to have something. I did not have enough faith to trust my baby to the universe, to chance.

Two months later, I heard a quavering voice on the local NPR affiliate as I drove home from work: "Because of our combined income level, we qualify for public assistance; so my baby's health insurance will be covered by Healthy Start. This means I'm a pregnant Medicaid recipient working on my second master's degree. I am deeply grateful for this public assistance but saddened and shocked that OSU is pushing this cost back onto the state welfare system." Oh, for God's sake . . . of all the hackneyed attempts to play on public sympathies. The clichéd trope of the helpless and great-with-child female.

The most nauseating part of the broadcast was that the voice was mine.

I stopped at a red light and reached over to shut off the radio. I closed my eyes and thought insanely, "How dare she?" By *she* I meant my evil exhibitionist twin.

There is obviously something suspicious about a woman who would write her most intimate details in essays and then try to get them printed so other people can read them. I honestly don't know what to make of someone who would also volunteer her belly and unborn fetus as a media visual in an activist campaign.

Somewhere in my head I do have a "normal" person upon whom the activist and the writer both feed in parasitic glee—and I let them, so it's entirely my own problem. At one of these cores, I am shy, if you will believe it. That sane and shy version of me drove home from the press conference, cringing at what I had just done.

A few weeks earlier, the graduate-student healthcare committee had asked for help finding speakers for their press conference on the problem of graduate health insurance. I volunteered. "Yeah, I know a pregnant chick who'd be perfect." As an organizer, I'd spent a decade prodding people to spill their personal stories into microphones. As a reporter, I'd scribbled those sentences into notebooks and slapped them into four-paragraph stories. But I'd never been a poster child myself. So I probably deserved it.

Ten people spoke at the press conference. Why did they have to pick my voice to broadcast? But I knew why: the belly is a great propaganda tool. It worked on the reporters. I knew it would. Would the bosses at my four jobs hate me or fire me? Maybe no one would hear the story.

At home Skate stood at the sink washing the wood dust from his hands. He dumped the dregs of coffee from his thermos into the sink. He turned around to look at me as if he were seeing me for the first time and was a little freaked out. His sweaty forehead was striped with construction grime.

"Damn," he said, "I heard you. You put it all out there . . . my name . . . what we make each month."

"Are you okay with that?" I asked. It was maybe a little late to ask permission.

The next morning, I leafed through the metro section of the *Columbus Dispatch* and prayed to the journalism gods. "Please, oh please, oh please," I whispered. "Let the story have gotten bumped. Let it be a tiny, one-inch blurb."

I flipped past a story about Arnold Schwarzenegger's ties to central Ohio and skimmed a feature about workers at a popcorn plant dealing with lung infections from an airborne chemical-butter cloud. Livestock prices, obituaries . . . almost home free.

I turned the last page. My own belly and boobs distended massively from the newsprint. I closed my eyes and moaned. The photo was huge, at least three inches tall. I forced myself to look: downcast eyes, Eastern European hawk's beak of a nose. "I want my healthcare!" A wash of olive skin and beige shirt . . . a brownout of maternal sadness, clutching a poster board scrawled with Magic Marker.

I held up the page for my husband to see and winced in disgust.

He scowled. "Wait," he asked, "why aren't you happy? Isn't this what you wanted?"

"I know," I said wearily. "It's a good thing." That was why I wanted to throw up.

I hauled my pregnant butt off the couch, and my fetus son ricocheted against my spine. I went upstairs to search for a maternity shirt that still fit me, steeling myself against a day of embarrassment. Everyone was going to think I was a whiner, a hysterical pregnant woman using her belly to get attention, a woman who couldn't get her shit together and should have just sucked it up and taken out a few more student loans, a social services parasite. My creative-writing colleagues had dedicated their lives to subtlety, for God's sake; and this was so . . . obvious.

Thankfully, none of my bosses fired me or ended my freelance contracts, and nobody called me a whiner within earshot. One office manager even stapled the picture and article to the staff bulletin board. I looked away whenever I passed it.

Although my sad face in newsprint implied that Medicaid was a kind of punishment, the state-run program with its faults still ranks as my fondest and sweetest healthcare memory. Among the ex-policies that have loved me and left me, this one still makes me smile at the effortless way I fell into its attentive and unconditional love. But I resisted that destiny, waited until I could not find any other partner before I backed into its embrace.

About a month before the press conference, nestled in a thick cloak of financial doom and self-castigation, I had discovered the Ohio social services Web site. I knew about it because I had covered this beat as a reporter and then used these sources as a health-care organizer. In some ways, the destination could not have been more obvious. I sorted through the fine print on the Healthy Start Web site and downloaded the simple application. I filled it out and mailed it with copies of our pay stubs. I waited for a form letter rejection that I imagined would instruct me to sell my remaining CDs to the music store and my semi-favorite clothes to the resale shop: "Come back when you're truly desperate and unable to fake it as middle-class."

A few weeks later, a computer-generated letter arrived to declare the fetus and me eligible for state benefits. The kid would be insured for his first year of life, and beyond that if my income stayed low enough. Other packets explained where to go for health exams. I even got to choose between the standard Medicaid or CareSource, a state-run HMO. I received a case number and a harried caseworker who returned my phone calls.

At the pharmacy a few weeks later, I waited for my first CareSource prescription, resting my hands on the shelf of my huge belly. The pharmacist smiled at me and handed me my health card and the paper bag containing my antibiotics.

"You're all set," she said.

I stood there. I held out my credit card.

"No, you're CareSource," she said. "You're all set. No charge."

No charge. Should I bolt for the door before she realized her mistake? Was this some sort of sick pharmacist humor? She held her perky grin, growing only a little impatient as she glanced at the long line of people waiting behind me.

No charge. Not $5, a nominal amount to remind me of my shameful dependence. Not $10.74, a faceless yet exact figure to convey my status as a field in a database. Not $179.00, the free-market cost on a credit card, a threat that the next illness might be the tilt in my financial pinball game.

Zero. Nothing. "Are you sure?" I asked.

She pushed the bag in my direction, maybe wondering whether she'd need to call security. "Have a good day," she said, and then turned to the person behind me.

Up until that point, the closest I'd come to an honest surge of adult patriotism was a warm glow of gratitude while sitting in a library or hiking through a state park. But when the accordion automatic doors opened and revealed the pharmacy parking lot, I wanted to go out and hug a mail carrier or state employee. I wanted to find a federal building and kiss its marble surface. I lumbered to my car, an intense heat fanning from my heart. I knew with my political mind that this whole problem—and the gratitude at being rescued from a small crisis—could have been solved with better legislation and a different healthcare model. But right then there was no room for anger in my pregnancy-squished brain, only a relief that extended far beyond the edges of my skin.

I can hardly describe the sidewalk that day, the blacktop. The streetlamps felt like mine; we were cousins. How can I explain this feeling of *belonging*? That day in the parking lot is a bubble of memory in smell and sunlight. The yellow lines had been freshly painted on to stark, rich black asphalt. Across the street, there was a thrift store that was moving to a new location, with large handwritten signs taped to the store windows advertising the new address. The dialysis center next door was under construction with scaffolding slanted against its orange stucco facade. The sun was out, the shafted midwestern light that goes in gold and yellow columns from behind tall cumulonimbus clouds.

And there I was, a soft and vulnerable body and bones, with a smaller body and bones inside. As I contained a fetus, I grew outward with layers from a history, growing up in public school where I ate waxy government cheese, driving on roads, playing in public parks, and benefitting in a trillion other ways from being a U.S. citizen even as I raged over the policies of our government. But I'd never before had the sense that a small piece of my future had been saved, that I had been plucked back from the edge of something bigger than I could handle or scavenge or duct tape or organize or rage against.

I was a U.S. citizen in the fullest sense of the phrase right then, a publicly funded construction project. It may be true that I have never felt as anonymously worthy, grateful, or cared about as I did right then. It didn't matter what I had scored on a test, what my résumé looked like, or what choices I had made. Despite everything, I was safe—unconditionally and without judgment.

I sat in my car and put my head on the steering wheel. I cried and cried, leaving a wet spot on the northern hemisphere of my belly.

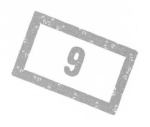

THE MELODRAMA DISCOUNT

My husband Skate clutched his abdomen and writhed on the vinyl stretcher in the ER holding area. A nurse came in, probed his middle, and said he probably had acute appendicitis. "They'll probably have to operate right away," she said.

She left. An hour passed.

I patted his forehead and said, "Don't worry," but the lobe of my brain devoted to healthcare finance churned in fear of the final price tag for this adventure. I dissociated into an explanation-of-benefits haze. The itemized bill—if it included the slitting open of guts, cleaning up of guts, and all those ER docs—would add up to thousands and thousands and thousands of dollars.

Two hours passed. I stood in the hallway of the triage area, hoping to flag down a nurse. The weight of my belly pulled at the ligaments around my hips, and I felt as if my hip bones and spine might burst into flames. I leaned against the metal doorjamb and tried to use my eyeballs as lasers to cut into the neck of the nurse who sat at a desk across from us, talking on the phone.

The nurse did not glance up when I started to keen and wipe my snot on my stretch maternity sleeve. Wet faced, I turned into the triage room. My husband shuddered feverishly, then leaned over and puked into a kidney-shaped plastic basin. If we were going to pay for every cent of this, the least they could do was fix him. I hung my head out the door and glared. I asked for water, for ice, for a clean puke bucket, hoping that my eye rolling would unjam this hospital deadlock.

Wearing a blue and purple low-cut paisley tunic over my hugely pregnant belly, I had braided a strand of hair on either side of my head into a hippie do and called myself Mama Cass. The Halloween party in 2003 was the week before Skate's hospital adventure; I'm pretty sure this was the first decent Halloween costume I'd ever come up with. The year before, I'd dressed up as a garage sale, with tags stuck all over me. That costume had required too much explaining.

My husband knocked on the door of his friend—Joe's house was a brick ranch in the neighborhood where the local alternative thirty-somethings were settling down and buying houses. You could walk the blocks of the university neighborhood and point out the gardens and lawns of this and that seminal punk band in Columbus, play connect-the-dots to trace musical influences and ex-loves and feuds and scenes, now all neighbors.

Joe opened the door, the delight on his face apparent as he bit back a grin and the crow's-feet wrinkled at the corner of his eyes. I saw him as one of the patron saints of our marriage, since he'd donated all the food for our wedding. He sized me up and said something like, "Jesus, you're about to pop."

Joe's new girlfriend, Heather, ushered us in past an elaborate tray of snacks in Halloween themes. After introductions, we were led out to a bricked patio, where I sat on a wooden patio bench and leaned back to take the pressure off my hips.

My husband sat next to me, and I reached for a forbidden pull from his beer. He surrendered the beer and glanced around at the crowd on the patio. "Damn, honey, cut it out. People are going to think you're a mess," he said.

I shrugged. "If any of these drunks want statistics on when a fetus is vulnerable to one sip of alcohol, I'll give them the most recent research." We were bantering, chatting: this was not a tense moment. And I felt too big to mess with. I knew trouble, and this was not it.

What I remember most from that night on the patio is the pinkish gold light of a late-fall midwestern evening (has light ever been lovelier anywhere, have clouds ever been so piled in Sistine stacks and curls?) with oak leaves above us and bugs buzzing and pricking at sweat-sticky skin. The guys holding brown beer bottles by their necks glanced sidelong at my husband, the way guys will size up a man who apparently has enough testosterone to get a woman that pregnant. At one point, I grabbed my husband's carpenter bicep and held it, needing that solid muscle. In feeling his arm I felt history. He'd known Joe since they were hell-bent teenagers, and Joe's past was as checkered and raw as my husband's. I knew about Joe's divorce and recent happiness with Heather, who was obviously trying very hard to win over Joe's friends in a sweet show of punk-rock domesticity.

"Here's to surviving our twenties," I wanted to say with that one sip of beer on a pink night. "Here's to getting knocked up and buying a cheap ranch house and making sandwiches shaped like spiders. Here's to hope."

In a flurry of sudden activity that must have been triggered by the flapping of a butterfly's wings in Madagascar, my husband was rolled from the ER triage holding area to a room with stretchers in rows. The beds were each enclosed in hanging curtains, and each holding bay had a little TV. Across a central hallway, a youngish man coughed disastrously. As often happens in the ER, the unavoidable details of his narrative filtered and mixed with ours.

"Sir, how long have you been coughing blood?" We could see and hear the coughing man across the room, and a nurse must have noticed us looking. She yanked the curtain closed, shielding us from the sight of each other but giving nobody any privacy.

"Well, I think it's about three years now," continued the cougher from behind the curtain. "But it seems to have just gotten really bad lately."

"What do you mean by 'bad?'"

"Like, it's just started to be a whole lot of blood."

There but for the grace of God go I, I thought to myself. It was only by chance or luck that I was not Blood Cougher's girlfriend or wife. Men are so Zen about their bodies, watching with bemused detachment as chunks of their insides come out and fall off. Balding—a natural, nonfatal process—was cause for alarm, but bona fide medical crises could be deferred.

A nurse gave Skate a big beaker of red fluid to drink, a contrast solution to make his intestines more visible for an MRI. As he gagged down the pitcher of lukewarm chemicals, we heard the Blood Cougher describe his daily smoking habit.

Even in that sweaty, painful mania, my husband met my eyes and smiled. Yes, his appendix might blow any moment, but at least we were "middle-class" in the whacked-out American definition of it: we would feel hopeful and empowered enough to seek help when coughing blood. We would sheepishly ask a doctor about a seeping, festering wound. Even as a low-income emergency, we could feel superior and almost of the country club set in comparison to someone who felt utterly unable to stop killing himself. My husband lay back for a moment and put the empty beaker on the bedside table. A second after he relaxed, he shot forward again and puked up the red fluid. The second beaker of fluid stayed in Skate's stomach long enough to perform the MRI.

After the test, a nurse wheeled Skate back to the ER holding area.

"My appendix is fine," he moaned, tossing his head back and

forth on the stretcher, skin sweaty and gray, eyes screwed tight. An appendectomy would have been comforting at this point.

The surgeon and the doctor stood above the stretcher and batted the possibilities back and forth: Ulcerative colitis? Crohn's disease? Cancer? This must be how doctors hone in on a family of conditions, working their way hand over hand from the tragic to the mundane; but I always feel obliged to imagine myself—or in this case, the father of my nearly born child—as beset by every disease they invoke.

A third doctor stepped into the curtained holding bay, holding a dark-filmed MRI image. "You haven't been shot recently, have you?" he asked.

Skate had never been shot, but we both recoiled as if just now feeling the bullet's entry.

"The test revealed what looks like a tiny bit of metal in your colon," said the film-reading doctor. Did my husband work with metal? Had he been in a car accident?

He *had* been to the dentist yesterday, he said.

"Ahh," said the doctor. He explained that a tiny bit of filling had probably fallen down my husband's throat and was passing through his system, a common occurrence.

"You mean the dentist did this to me?" Skate asked, feverishly looking for someone human-sized to blame, out of his head, still stuck on the bullet-wound scenario.

"Hmmm," said the doctor. "No, it's unlikely that a bit of filling would cause this."

Skate was finally admitted to the hospital and sent up to a room while the surgeons continued to watch him in order to decide what to do about his guts. An IV pumped antibiotics into his huge carpenter's veins, and he miserably chewed on ice chips and tightened his fists. "That fucking dentist. As soon as I get out of here, I'm going to sue the shit out of him," he said from his hospital bed.

Skate's dental ire made more sense in context. The dentist was actually a dental student in the low-income clinic at Ohio State University School of Dentistry. A year earlier, Skate and I had been gamely enthusiastic about the prospect of discount dental care, despite the fact that I had had my own bad experiences in the past. We were both so cheap and poor, and dental care was so expensive, that our optimism blurred any fear about pain or mistakes.

After three or four uneventful but long visits, he had been offered an opportunity that made both of us very happy: he had an unusual and challenging configuration of decay on one of his teeth. He could serve as a live test subject for the dental student's board certification exam. He would be paid for his time and his mileage to and from Cleveland. And on top of it all, the filling would be free. It was like winning the lottery! We might have wondered at that point whether it would be a good idea to submit to a dental student working in a high-stakes, live-testing environment with an audience. But we did not.

Sometime during the filling of this challenging and special cavity, Skate felt the searing pain of a dental error. This was confirmed a few hours later when he was sent home with an apology and the carbon copy of a certificate for a free round of treatment for whatever mistakes might have been committed. "It looks like I pulped the tooth," said the friendly and regret-filled dentist. "Pulped," when describing oranges, might sound as if the entity in question was thrown into a food processor and liquefied. With teeth, *pulped* means that a dentist went too deep in pursuing decay and made contact with the root, thus exposing it to the air, in which case the tooth would most likely require either a crown or a root canal. We then embarked on a saga of collecting receipts in a manila folder and screaming at the dental billing office when they proceeded to send us exorbitant bills for the repair of the pulped tooth. We saved the bills in a manila folder and began the time-consuming process of documenting and replying to each bill, copying and sending the note from the dental student claiming responsibility for the mistake.

And now Skate's insides rebelled for no reason the doctors could see. When my husband slept, I pregnantly shuffled up and down the dimly lit halls, which were painted in shades of internal-organ gray. Moans echoed from rooms with half-open doors. Braxton Hicks prelabor contractions rippled up and down my belly, and my son bore down on the base of my spine. To distract myself, I waddled down to the charity-care office to get an application for financial assistance. Tear-streaked face, pregnant belly . . . believe me, I played it up for all it was worth, hoping there would be an extra discount for melodrama.

I got out my cell phone and called relatives who owed me for years of their nuttiness. My calling list included people whom I knew to be emotionally empty wells incapable of empathy, and they were nice and very sympathetic and worried I was going to anxiety attack myself into labor.

"I guess it would be convenient if you had the baby," one of them said. "You're already in the hospital."

The pink warmth of last week's Halloween-party evening had disappeared, and the appropriate November midwestern sheet of gray slid in to take its place. I drove home alone one evening to get magazines, underwear, and socks for my husband; and as I returned that night, something about the hospital parking gate made me cry. The wooden arm, striped with caution colors of black and yellow, raised in an arc like a rifle, as if to let me into danger because I had reached the required level of hazard.

Gray cement walls of the hospital parking garage. White cement of the hospital where I'd visited a friend after her birth, where I'd attended childbirth classes, now shrouded in fog. The maze of curbs and Do Not Enter signs and arrows leading me back into the hospital's hive felt needlessly obtuse. The car felt huge and metal and dangerous; I could barely turn the steering wheel, and yet there was no choice but to continue with all of these trajectories: toward birth, toward death.

This was exactly what *wife* meant, apparently: pregnant, alone, navigating concrete barriers, carrying a plastic shopping bag full of clothes, attempting to dredge up encouragement, and waiting to cry by myself out in the overwaxed linoleum hallway that glared like a headache. Yet there was comfort here, in the nonthought of doing these necessary tasks: I was being tested. This was being a wife, and I was doing it.

Happily, I did not go into labor. Skate graduated from ice chips to Jell-O. After a day and a half of blood tests, the doctors declared that some sort of bacteria was the culprit of his ailment and that there were a few possible causes. One was the student dental clinic itself—maybe the equipment had been improperly sterilized. Another chief suspect was my husband's carpentry job that week: in the process of rehabbing an apartment, he had needed to rip up a large section of a wood floor that had been soaked with dog urine. At this point, the source didn't matter. Three days later, he began to feel better and was discharged with a diagnosis of bacterial colitis.

Two weeks after that, in November 2003, my little progeny decided he was ready to see the world, two weeks ahead of schedule. My water broke and I was shipped off to the maternity ward, where I presented a birth plan like the ones I'd read about in the pregnancy books. That plan got folded up and crumpled in a bag, along with scented lotion and CDs and other ridiculousness, the first moment a contraction barreled over me like a locomotive. Then the contractions stopped.

I was tied to a bunch of monitors but had this weird feral instinct that if I could walk and go someplace quiet and dark, away from the fluorescent glare and beeping of the hospital room, I could start regular labor. They let me walk a bit but then gave me a drug to hasten labor, followed by an epidural.

And my son did his job, arriving in network—a normal delivery. The grand total for the obstetrical mess and hospitality came to $300, truly a good deal for a new human being. I held him and made friends with the Healthy Start woman who came to visit. I called the breast-feeding consultant from the hospital phone and couldn't reach her, so I called from an outside line and left voice mails until someone appeared at my door to help me with nipples and holds and lactation whatnot. My new son was my most important health insurance–organizing project. Even if he was getting free care, it would be the best care I could get him.

The invoice for Skate's three-day hospital stay came to more than $8,000. This—to my joy—activated his sleeping-giant catastrophic health policy, which coughed up $5,000 and earned me a rueful and grateful, "Always listen to the wife."

The good news was that we saved $5,000. But we were still deep in trouble and $3,000 in the hole. "We" were a semi-employed and still-weak carpenter who could only eat toast and mashed potatoes, an unemployed proofreader who was on leave from graduate school without maternity benefits, and an infant who was just now winding up into the beginning stages of colic. Add a midwestern winter to this mix, and you have a cocktail of ear-shattering desperation.

I attacked the problem of the nonexistent $3,000 with the full force of my postpartum hormonal being. The great thing was that our previously low income now looked ridiculous on the charity-care application, so our baby was already pulling his weight. I added extensive handwritten notes in the small comment field to explain our situation. The hysterical comments overflowed the boxes and crept up the margins back toward the top of the page.

A few weeks after we submitted the paperwork, Skate got a call from the hospital. Standing in the kitchen, he clutched the phone to his face and said "uh-huh" as he listened. His eyes scanned my face with urgency and shock. I whispered hoarsely in a kind of mimed scream, "Is it your doctor?"

He hung up, and I forced myself to breath. He put his hand on the counter.

"What?" I said finally.

"They wrote it all off," he said.

"What?"

It wasn't the doctor. It was the billing department of Riverside Hospital, which had processed our application and forgiven the entire $3,000 we owed them.

I dropped to my knees on the kitchen floor. It sounds too dramatic now, and I have seen this image in fiction: "She dropped to her knees." I didn't exactly feel faint; it wasn't as though my knees buckled. Instead, my tight shoulders and knotted hamstrings, my clenched stomach muscles, all loosened momentarily with a flood of relief and gratitude. I knelt and touched the rough wood floor, the one we'd discovered beneath layers of linoleum and glue. Don't imagine a lovely, shining wood floor like those in an interior decorating magazine. The old wood planks dipped with triangular gouges from the scraper. They were grayish, coated with a layer of dust and gummy residue from a coat of polyurethane that hadn't dried properly. The floor had gaps and holes in it. Don't imagine a kitchen the way you've seen a kitchen shine. Imagine a kitchen made from wood my husband salvaged from construction jobs and dumpsters. In that kitchen, $3,000 meant a quarter of a year's worth of wages.

I knelt on the floor and cried. My two-month-old son was asleep in his bassinette, and those $3,000 were his. I felt as though I, too, could curl up and sleep in the in-box on the desk of the charity-care office at Riverside Hospital, in a quiet and white space as shaded and bleak as the sky outside. I wanted the cheek of a billing-department clerk to kiss. Poverty and numbers alone had run us up against a last refuge, the generosity of a hospital that could write us off by claiming a donation to the poor. These things are the opposite of a guarantee and so the opposite of a sense of security. They impart the adrenaline rush of a bullet whizzing by one's ear, clipping millimeters of flesh and delivering a narrow margin of safety that emphasizes its own transience. This was my first real sense of us as three, as a family: three was the number that made our combined income not genteel poverty but a bit of an emergency, and three was the number that made the $3,000 disappear. I felt so guilty for putting my son to work in the numbers game in the weeks before he even understood the outlines of this world. He was already working, already helping with too much of the burden, for this thin-stretched family. Our lack—our inability to meet his needs—had taken care of that baby when I couldn't. I had to promise myself that after this moment, such a blessing would never happen again.

In one of her columns in the *Nation*, Katha Pollitt wonders whether universal healthcare is the ultimate family value. She examines the statistics of "divorce as triggered by the financial and emotional stresses of uninsured illness" and contemplates the shared costs on an entire family when one member has chronic and untreated health problems, ranging from less money for soccer camp all the way to personal bankruptcy, reminding readers that half of the personal bankruptcies in this country are sparked in part by medical bills.

It would take five years for my divorce from Skate to be finalized in 2009, and I would never claim that money or its lack caused the demise of our marriage. But I knew that money could exhaust a man and a woman, could take the energy required to feed love, to raise a child. I continue to believe that love can grow where money cannot. But worry is a knife. You watch the blade. Tensing against that knife-edge takes the attention and focus that might have gone to your family.

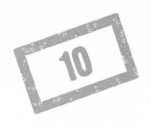

HEALTHY START

I nursed my son Ivan around the clock, it seemed; I spent so much time staring at his tiny folded ear as he lay in my lap that I became fascinated with the ear's structure and its lovely whorls. When he napped, I looked up the names of the curves, each designed to focus and amplify sound: the outer rim of the helix, the inner nub of the tragus, and the curved cave of the cymba conchae. I had grown that pink ear from molecules. My body was food, water, shelter, comfort, and meaning as his brain unfolded. In Maslow's hierarchy of needs, the supporting layers of the pyramid ascend toward the point, getting smaller and smaller as the biological need is differentiated from, and yet serves as the foundation for, social needs such as contact, accomplishment, and self-actualization.

How does one pyramid support and grow another? Surely the tiny triangle is not balanced precariously on its mother's point. Maybe I took off my top layers, putting them aside like a hat, to grow my miniature pyramid. Or maybe a pyramid is too simple a structure to describe a mother and her baby.

Even in the gray wash of sleep deprivation, sometimes forgetting to eat, nursing and nursing, I could ascend briefly past the base of my own pyramid to reach Maslow's fifth level (cognitive fulfillment, the need to understand) or even the sixth (aesthetic, the appreciation and search for beauty, balance, and form). As a mother it could not be otherwise. I reached up into awe and then slipped back down my own slanted surface, sometimes venturing down below basic needs into the catacombs, the substructure of worry where the dead and the powdery past are kept.

The Ohio Department of Job and Family Services sent me a humble notice on rough paper. "You and your infant qualify for the following benefits: food aid for moms with young children (WIC) and the state-funded health program. If at any time you are found to exceed the preset income levels, you will be disenrolled. You will need to recertify every three months."

A public health nurse came to visit and glanced around our house in a practiced scan. Her job must have required her to check for warning signs: a drugged-out mom, a sagging floor or freezing house, or a lack of food. She smiled brightly to see the obvious needs met. She explained that I would need to schedule quarterly visits with the state clinic to get checkups. I could also send in proof of periodic immunizations for a series of $25 gift cards to the local grocery store. I listened, fully focused, waiting to follow any instructions. I wanted any task they would give me.

I had always finished to-do lists, but the rewards had never seemed so immense. These tasks would give us life. They would give us food. There was no complex emotional price to pay, no gauntlet of shame or public ridicule. They demanded no skin to mark with the stripes of scars. They made me sign no form attesting to my sin or promising never to be so stupid again. She smiled at me, and this is the moment I will always remember as a bureaucracy showing me the meaning of unconditional love. All you need is need itself, and I will give you peanut butter in return.

She gave me a canvas tote bag filled with a free blanket, a cloth teddy bear, and books on infant development. She placed my pink, squirming, floppy boy on a portable scale, supporting his head as he cried at the unfamiliar touch of cold metal on his skin.

Abraham Maslow, who created the pyramid describing levels of need and fulfillment, drew his theories from his own life stresses. He was the eldest of seven children born in Brooklyn to Jewish parents who had emigrated from Russia. Without formal education themselves, his mother and father pushed him forward in schooling. Imagine him at home tripping over more and more siblings and babies in a crowded apartment. Maslow transformed personal crisis directly into his scholarly agenda, saying at one point, "I was awfully curious to find out why I didn't go insane." Biographies describe Maslow as "very lonely as a boy," a boy who "found his refuge in books."

I also found refuge for my family in text. I worked as a medical proofreader on ingredient labels for chemo drugs and on instruction manuals for IV pumps, wrote freelance articles for local magazines, and judged a feature-writing contest for a horse racing magazine. I taught a college journalism course and worked as a part-time publicity intern. I finished my thesis for graduate school. I submitted applications for post–grad school jobs.

I tried to work while nursing, folding a page over a book and leaning to the left while he nursed at the right. I tucked pens in books and pages to mark my place when he woke and screamed with colic. I lost the loop of text and hungered for the alphabet, afraid I would never get it back. My son must have absorbed that hunger and fear from the pores of my skin in microscopic letters.

I cried at stoplights and while washing bottles. I picked up a flyer for a local moms' group and cried when I read that it was for stay-at-home moms. I did not stay at home; my clearest memories from those months took place in my car. I bought a car cigarette-lighter adapter for my breast pump. I wheeled around Columbus on the I-270 beltway, holding the steering wheel with one hand while the other hand squashed the breast pump nozzle under my shirt.

After a month or two of weeping, I made an appointment in winter 2004 with my psychiatrist in the university medical complex. I did not waste time with complex strands of emotion.

"Look," I said, "I think I have postpartum. I can't stop crying." I explained that I was waiting for recertification for prescription benefits now that my son had been born. I had been bounced from benefits because I'd made some money doing freelance writing, and I had taken myself off the university plan to save money. "I can't afford to pay for a prescription even if you give me one."

The psychiatrist tapped at his laptop and pulled up the latest research on my antidepressant. He explained the comparatively low rate of transfer into breast milk, the research on infant brain development, and bioaccumulation of serotonin reuptake inhibitors. My working dose had always been low; the potential effect on my son was minimal, especially when you considered suicide as the alternative.

"I know what we can do," said the quiet doctor with his thinning hair and glasses, his flannel shirt. He left his office for a moment. I closed my eyes, listening to the fountain in the corner.

He opened the door holding a handful of sample bottles of my old antidepressant, the sky blue friend I hadn't needed at all during pregnancy. He handed me a form from the drug manufacturer. I was to state my income, to fill it out before I left; he'd fax it in that afternoon. Before I left his office, I swallowed a sky blue pill at the drinking fountain in the hallway.

Maslow's seventh layer is self-actualization, which includes the need to reach potential and to seek "peak experiences." That peak at the water fountain with cold water and the chalky nudge of a pill in my throat was an inverted summit, a divot in the earth that nonetheless altered my course.

The peak cleared any visions of motherhood as pink and pastel blue clouds. Instead, I saw my raw materials—my personality and my resources—like a handful of pills, just beans, not magic anymore, not limitless. The choices lay behind me: the option to worry without action, to hang back in shame, or to turn away from begging and dependence. I have never been so needy nor so proud to take care of myself. I learned that motherhood was the point of a dull-edged, stainless steel tool, polished and ready for use, the surrender to a larger genetic will to survive.

I lugged Ivan's awkward car seat into the St. Stephen's Community Clinic for my first WIC appointment. They would check to make sure Ivan was growing, and then they would give us food coupons and reapprove health benefits. He napped, leaving a quarter-sized wet spot of drool on the cushioned headrest.

I flinched as I signed in, waiting for them to look in a file and tell me there'd been a mistake and that I would not get access. I had dressed consciously for this visit. I wore the kind of cardigan sweater, hoop earrings, and clogs that whispered "college girl." I'd always been good at scavenging primo finds from garage sales and Goodwill; I had expensive tastes that led me to the best fabrics amid the hushed *click-click-click* of women sliding hangers on thrift-store racks to sort among the rows as they collected their harvests of cast-off clothes.

They called my name, opened the door, and directed me to a room.

I chatted with the caseworker and the nurse and thanked each profusely. They took my blood and my weight, then my son's. I sat on the plastic chair in the examining room, holding Ivan tightly as if we'd just gotten on the merry-go-round at the fair. "Look!" I wanted to wave to invisible spectators. "It's starting! It's working! Healthcare!"

The doctor recorded my baby's growth and handed me coupons

for beans and cheese and milk. They offered a free breast pump, training on child care, and a hotline phone number especially for breast-feeding questions. I held in my hand a reminder card for my next appointment. In my pocket, I tucked prescriptions for an antibiotic for me and ear drops for him. Gratitude warmed me and held me. I asked about spitting up and about sleep, and each question came out in a half laugh of disbelief.

We used the milk coupons gratefully and wished there were coupons for vegetables, rice, or meat. The veggie coupons to the farmers' markets wouldn't be available until early summer. Instead, our coupon packets contained vouchers for a hefty supply of dried pinto beans, tuna, and peanut butter. I went to the grocery in our neighborhood, where the clerks whipped through the WIC transaction without batting an eye. In the grocery stores of the nicer neighborhood near campus, I learned my vouchers would deadlock a checkout line endlessly as the clerk puzzled over some code, voided and voided a transaction, then yelled to a supervisor, "Can you help me with this WIC coupon?" as my face got hot.

I want to write that I got over the shame, because my brain disapproves. Do I think I'm too good to be poor? The shame turned me inside out and shifted me slightly, revealing my prejudices like a strobe light catching me in an awkward pose. It was a good thing to stand in that checkout line, watching the black rubber belt roll onward and onward forever toward the cash register.

Each victory in this new world of want and mothering was more than mere domestic work, the foraging and gathering of berries and seeds. It was like sprinting on powerful legs to hunt a wooly mammoth. I wrestled and won things I did not believe I could catch.

Each dot matrix income verification form asked me how much money I earned in the previous twelve weeks. I had to be careful. If I earned too much, I would lose benefits. The real threat was the large gray area: above poverty level but far below enough money to buy the cheapest health insurance. I shuffled numbers and jobs to calculate a passage between those narrow rocks toward safety. When I summon moments from my son's first year, the chest-clench and the heart-stop feelings involve paperwork—forms and blank lines. Somewhere buried between the memories of rough paper and a mantra said slowly and carefully into a caseworker's voice mails is the touch of my son's infinitely soft cheek against my lips and the smell of him—fresh skin and rainwater.

I remember, too, the frantic, sweaty panic of his crying from colic; the wrestling to breast-feed the active, flailing baby who was already wiry and athletic, primed for motion; the exhausting struggle with the awkward plastic car seat bump-bumping against my calf as I balanced it against the weight of my labor-activism folders and binders in a bag hanging from my other shoulder.

Ivan's first labor rally was that spring, and he looked on in bright-eyed wonder above the quilted edge of the carrier strapped to my front. I bobbed up and down in time to a beat from a bass drum as noise ricocheted off the glass windows of the buildings downtown. Purple-shirted organizers and labor activists, including janitors who cleaned the buildings around us, yelled and shook soda cans filled with beans and rocks.

The janitors, mostly Somali immigrants, worked for various third-party contractors. One boss had threatened to fire a man who stayed home to help his wife after the birth of their third child. He went back to work, and his wife's middle split open along the stitched-up caesarian wound as she bent to lift up one of her other young children. This was the kind of horror story we told at every press conference, but the reporters told us the stuff was too depressing, not sexy enough. So this news rarely made it into the paper.

On May 18, 2004, Ivan turned six months old. The lilacs popped in purple fireworks, and the river and rain brought forth green from the muck and bark. We took a walk down by the Olentangy River; he was slung in front of me in the blue quilted carrier. He gnawed on the fabric in front of his face, soaking it with baby spit, the white dome of his hairless head bobbing like a buoy atop the blue fabric.

Ivan began meeting my eyes with sparks of laughter, with a complex and delightful sense of humor, comic timing in his arched eyebrows and his gummy laughter. The gush of breast-feeding had slackened as he began to eat solid food, and colic was behind us. His basic needs were met. His busy brain was working and building; the coos and hand flops assimilated themselves in a cluster of gestures and half words that began to make language. He could sit, reach for things, and watch the world's motion and blobs of color as his eyes sparked. Like two ballroom dancers, or like a setter and a spiker on a volleyball team, we had reached the hum of comfort and shared purpose that is a kind of God to me. I caught the rhythm of mothering, finally—yes, I can pack a bag and clean a diaper and drink coffee and even laugh. The dark winter had driven me into a blank place and a need that required clearing. I had begun meditating every day and had joined a Tibetan Buddhist temple.

Mothering changes the mother's brain as well as the child's. The extraordinary demands of multitasking called for a reknitting of my neural networks. That hurts when it's happening, like an immersion course in a foreign language. To handle the frenzy, I needed focus and clarity. I needed the mental muscle to aggressively push aside the worry that had always picked at my mind. I set my sights on gratitude, on the gifts that came our way. Gratitude was not a pink cloud. It was a splintering piece of waterlogged lumber that kept us afloat. It was a rusty iron handhold. It was the raw material of safety.

Ivan cried stuffily and tugged at his pink ear. I took his temperature and found that he was running a slight fever. Worried that he had another ear infection, I called the pediatrician to make an emergency Saturday appointment.

"I'm sorry, ma'am," said the receptionist. "You have an outstanding balance, so that will need to be paid before you can be seen."

Oh no, oh no, oh no. Beneath the crepe paper of panic, though, I felt the lumber and rebar of motherhood's focus. I sighed, and it was a weighty sigh, like a sumo wrestler settling into battle with all the time in the world.

"I know what is happening," I said. I explained to the receptionist that the pediatrician's office kept submitting their bills to CareSource with codes that the state agency did not like. I had to nudge the process along by telling the billing woman how to code the medical procedures and by pointing out to her what had worked last time. The latest huge bill for a normal round of vaccinations had already been denied and resubmitted.

"Well, ma'am, that may be true," said the receptionist, "but the billing office is closed today, so I can't verify that."

I held Ivan against me, his face warm against my neck. He fussed and rubbed his nose in my hair. "I can't afford to pay for a load of vaccinations just so I can wait six months to get that money refunded," I said, a sharpness in my voice that I knew wouldn't help. I asked to be transferred to a nurse, who checked the same database screen, saw the same outstanding balance, and sadly reported I couldn't make an appointment unless I paid. I could take my son to Urgent Care, she said.

"Wait, wait—don't hang up," I said. I felt guilty, as though I was trying to swindle her into buying a set of knives she didn't need. A feverish clarity narrowed my vision, and I switched to bargaining mode. "Okay, let me ask you this: is it okay to wait for a few days with a possible ear infection?"

"Well, I can't really say without seeing him," she said, her voice trailing upward in doubt. I saw my loophole.

"Hmmm," I said. "All right. Imagine I had a son—in Canada, I guess—with a hypothetical ear infection. What would my options be, hypothetically?" I asked.

Far away in Canada, where an imaginary nurse would see my imaginary son, I got a hypothetical answer. "I can tell you this," she said, finally understanding what I wanted and what she could give. "Many parents do choose to wait a few days before starting antibiotics for an ear infection. I can tell you that much."

We waited out the weekend. After a pointed and relentless series of sumo-wrestling conversations with the billing office, I got the bill recoded, the charges paid, my office visit, and Ivan's antibiotics.

What's interesting now to me is the way in which Medicaid and the insurance system had trained me to see these challenges with new eyes. I still tensed with each new battle. My heart still whammered in my chest as I patted Ivan's back and punched the buttons on the phone with a rush that no caffeinated beverage could give me. But here's the thing: I no longer assumed this invoice, this number, this billing issue was correct. I had learned, I see now, that the system itself was irrational, logically inconsistent, and that if I went into it with a bit of logic and a bit of force, I already had the upper hand.

On June 24, 2004, I got a phone call from the pediatrician's office. The billing woman told me that all the charges we'd racked up on Medicaid since Ivan's birth—a grand total of about $1,500 to keep a very healthy baby that way—had been revoked. Medicaid had the power to reach into the doctor's bank account and take the money back. And it had.

Hands shaking, I called the CareSource office in tears, understanding even as I whipped myself into hysteria that this hysteria was functional, rational, and tactical. This was no time to be polite, and yelling was going to be completely necessary and completely called for. I did not waste time with the niceties; the first live human I reached got the complete level of my rage.

"Oh jeez," said the operator. "You're not the first one this has happened to." Lesson two—any human with a bit of empathy will inadvertently hand over valuable pieces of information to help reveal an underlying pattern.

The operator transferred me to someone who could see my screen in the database, and voice number two explained some snafu about previous health insurance eligibility on a form. I had to prove all over again that I'd been eligible for Medicaid. Voice number two transferred me to the voice mail of my case manager, my third one in nine months.

"This is an emergency. I will not talk to a voice mail. I need a return phone call immediately." I channeled my mom and every sharp-toned German-woman ancestor to rip into that recording.

I held Ivan on my hip as I trapped the phone receiver between ear and shoulder, leaving one hand free to rifle through my folder of forms and benefits statements. His concerned face, crumbled at the edges, was brave and solemn. God knows what fixation on which of Maslow's levels I imprinted on him that day.

Assuming my case manager would not call back fast enough—another functional assumption—I made myself into a crisis for the CareSource system. CareSource made me into the woman who was able to do that, and it was another transformation for which I am forever grateful. I had been hesitant to yell at these women—always women—because I had been a social worker. I knew they were ridiculously overworked and usually enraged at the system in which they worked. I knew they were not the roots of the problem, but they were the only branches of the problem I could reach.

I spoke to a woman who told me to fax my income verification forms to her supervisor, Stephanie.

"She's good," said the woman about Stephanie. "She doesn't misplace paperwork," as if this quality of Stephanie were an extra bonus, an above- and-beyond quality. I asked the woman how I could call to make sure that the fax had been received and processed.

"Just call and ask for Stephanie the supervisor," said the woman.

After I had gathered and faxed the next day, I called the switchboard and learned that Supervisor Stephanie didn't work there anymore.

My caseworker Lucy, called me two weeks later to tell me I needed to fax her a signed letter from my husband's boss on letterhead, along with my notice of severance from Ohio State, within two days. This last-minute documentation had been a hassle to collect the first time; now, with an infant, it became a sweaty mad dash, a mix of Kafka and Sesame Street.

For my next WIC recertification and checkup, I lugged Ivan to the door of St. Stephen's Clinic and read the sign taped to the glass door. The WIC office had been moved ten miles north to Morse Road, in the ground floor of an office complex. I drove fifteen minutes and found a pandemonium akin to the first day of third grade.

The lobby, built to contain only chairs and a few fake plants, had paper arrows pointing right (to the TB clinic) and left (to Prenatal). Patients wandered the hallways, trying to make sense of the arrows pointing in various directions like a treasure map.

I followed the arrows and asked the clerk why I hadn't received a notice about the clinic's address change. She took me back to a stack of bundled letters and rifled through a pile of alphabetized envelopes.

"I'm sorry this place is a mess," she said. "We got combined with another clinic, for efficiency or something like that." Miraculously, she plunged her hand in and located a crumpled envelope. She handed it to me. It was the missing income verification form, addressed to me, that had sparked the sucking of $1,500 from my doctor's bank account.

I studied it. "That's my address," I scowled. "Everything's correct."

She shrugged. "Well, for some reason it was returned. I wonder why." She asked if I still needed the form.

"No," I said. "I got it figured out."

July 22 was a day of freebies in our household. The mailman delivered a coupon for a free pair of cotton underwear from Victoria's Secret. A morning visit to the WIC office netted me coupons for fresh organic vegetables from the farmer's market. I was going to be Carrie Bradshaw eating a yuppie salad.

I buckled Ivan into his stroller, and we cruised around the stalls at the farmer's market. He murmured in glee to see the fresh red, orange, and yellow peppers on a table. A sign taped to a tarp said, "We take WIC coupons."

I pointed at a sheaf of organic corn. The young man bagged my corn, took my coupons, and said, "Have a great day!" No consternation, no confusion, and no looks up-and-down to imagine how I'd landed myself in whatever mess led to WIC.

Then we drove to Easton Towne Center, a "lifestyle mall" where we could look at the splashing fountain and I could use my coupon for free underwear. We strolled through the Aveda store so I could smell the potions and sip iced organic green tea from a paper cup. Ivan started to bat at the aromatherapy vials, so I awkwardly wheeled my tank of a stroller out into the sunlight.

Over at Victoria's Secret, I found the table with cotton panties and read the fine print to see which colors I could choose from. It was true: no purchase required. A clerk wrapped the undies in pink tissue paper and put them into a little pink paper tote with black corded handles. I liked the little bag almost more than the underwear, and I put it in the carrier underneath the stroller seat.

Ivan and I stopped at a bench outside in the shade so I could feed him some star-shaped wheaty snacks that liquefied like glue and stuck to everything as soon as they came into contact with baby spit. As I was trying to wrestle the wet wipes out of the diaper bag, a young man holding a clipboard stopped in front of us.

"Hi!" he said brightly. "I'm trying to sell magazine subscriptions to raise money for a trip to Italy to train for a broadcasting position with the BBC. I'm going there with my fiancée"—shoving a snapshot in my face, pulling it away—"and I only have three left to go for today. Can you help me out?"

I looked up at his face. His eyebrows seemed to have been tweezed or waxed badly, and his skin had the orangey tinge of a tanning booth or fake tanner. "I'm sorry," I said, "I don't think so." I pulled Ivan's sticky fingers from my hair.

"Look, I just need two minutes of your time. I have ADHD and I'm not on my medication right now. I need you to rate my communication skills so I can get the points I need." He didn't explain who would give him these points or what they meant. "Okay, can you give me a high five?" He held up his palm expectantly.

"Umm, whatever," I said. I tapped his palm with mine. "I have to go, I think. I need to change my son's diaper." I imagined the training he must have been given: get the customer to hold the card, get them to say yes, get them to shake hands or make physical contact.

"You seem like a nice person," he said. "Can you just look at this list of magazines?" He held in front of me a laminated card with names of expensive glossy publications.

"No," I said, "I'm sorry." I handed back the card.

"I'm sure you can afford it," he said. He ruffled pink carbon copies from his clipboard. "Look, I just need three more tonight. My birthday is in two weeks and I'm supposed to go to Italy."

"I can't," I said, a little alarmed as I shoved wipes and snacks roughly into pockets of the diaper bag. "It's not in my budget. I have to leave."

His tone turned harsh, and he gestured beneath the stroller. "You've been shopping here. You can afford a magazine subscription."

"No, I can't," I said. I put Ivan in the seat and buckled the plastic straps across his belly. Then jerking the stroller around the young man, I started to walk away.

"What, are you on welfare or something? It's not like you're on food stamps," he yelled after me.

I paused and turned. "I am on welfare, actually," I said, my voice shaking.

He looked me up and down, narrowing his eyes. "No you're not. Why would you come here? This is the fourth-wealthiest shopping mall in the country. You don't come here to walk around. You come here to shop. I can't believe you'd lie about something like that. You have money. You're not on welfare. I can't believe you'd lie—you're a mother with a baby and you're going to raise your kid to be a liar."

I walked away quickly, pushing the stroller, my body vibrating with fear at the brush with craziness. He stood behind me on the sidewalk, muttering "Bitch" among other choice phrases.

I wanted out of his line of sight. If he saw me go into a store, he'd think I was shopping, and then he'd feel in his insane head that he was right. Then I noticed that thought and made myself go into Anthropologie, an upscale store selling shabby-chic summer dresses and knickknacks. I wheeled the stroller deep into the protective waves of pink and sea green garments. I stopped in front of a display of $8 latte bowls, and then wheeled around the aisles and pulled Ivan's pink fingers away from the breakables, until I was sure the young man was gone.

Free stuff continued to find us, and I began to walk straight into offices with shoulders squared and my hand extended. I'm not sure if I learned this through Medicaid or through mothering. Both forces showed me how my young needed to be protected: with an agile and ready body and with free-swinging, well-aimed hands directed by a focused and calm mind. Each problem fixed, each real need of this tiny person attended to, each checkup with weight gain, each developmental milestone, and each kiss of healthy pink skin infused me with a sense that security could also be built and gained.

When Ivan was nine months old in summer 2004, the pediatrician tsked over Ivan's still-blocked and goopy left tear duct. He went over the benefits of a minor surgery now versus a major one later, and his billing office called CareSource to get the surgery authorized.

The nurses in the surgeon's office wrapped Ivan's arms and legs in a tight papoose of white bandages to keep him still. I leaned over the table, pressing his little body down as he writhed. They dabbed on a local anesthetic and then punctured the tiny membrane that would produce tears. I left the surgeon's office gasping, my arms quivering around him. My brave boy whimpered and his eyes drained blood, but he was already smiling, gumming my shoulder. His pink hand clutched an orange plastic dinosaur the nurse had given him.

On June 8, 1970, Maslow died of a heart attack at sixty-two, and one biographer describes him as having "years of ill health" before his death. I wonder about the toll that his personal stresses had on his body and his health. Stress led Maslow beyond Freud's exploration of hidden drives and Skinner's mapping of behavioral impulses. His "third force" theory was built around the question of motivation, or in his words, how people find the ability to not go insane. He revised his pyramid late in life, adding an eighth level: transcendence, or the need to help others achieve self-actualization. Maslow survived, I think, by building pyramids, these monuments to the third force, which keeps us going and urges us to help each other.

In a playgroup gathering, the mothers traded data about our babies' weights, the slobber bath of teething, and which kids got fussy and feverish after getting their shots. We built Maslow's third layer, belonging, out of Cheerios; we traded phone numbers scrawled on slips of paper, and plastic shopping bags filled with folded, laundered onesies and T-shirts.

I shared the latest news I learned from my friend Kathy about a state waiver for prekindergarten and daycare based on income. Kathy was thankfully two years ahead of me, passing down tricks like hand-me-downs. She had finally gotten her own house and was working in the healthcare industry without benefits, hoping and nudging her career toward coverage for herself and her kids.

One cute mom—a former performance poet who had red-dyed hair and hip-hugger jeans—gave a wry smile I recognized. She said she was waiting to schedule a checkup until baby's dad found a job. She shrugged with the complex acceptance an outsider takes for apathy.

I asked, in a whisper, "Have you heard of Healthy Start?"

"No," she said. Her eyebrows knit, and a rush of blood made a lacework pattern on the pink of her cheeks. That was the blush I'd seen before. I had previously assumed it was shame, but I saw it now for what it was: avid need and focus.

A lesbian mom, tattooed and pierced, cleared her throat, jiggled her toddler on her knee. "We're on it. It covers practically every doctor visit for Caleb. It's actually . . . great."

The tips and secrets poured out like a Tupperware party in reverse.

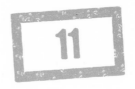

FRINGE BENEFITS

My son Ivan grew and thrived despite the invisibility of a foundation beneath him, like the game at the children's museum we visited in downtown Columbus where colored foam balls floated and spun, suspended by puffs of air. I was working in the summer of 2004 as a publicity intern for less than it cost me to put gas in my car and pay for childcare. In paying for the privilege of working, I saw each slim entry on my résumé as a hop toward stability, like playing a Frogger video game in which a happy little reptile dodges screaming traffic.

Paying to work pulled my checkbook closer to zero, the numbers buoyed a bit by part-time proofreading and freelance writing. I applied for an adjunct position to teach a few writing classes to engineering students at Ohio State. When they called to offer me the job, I did something on my own behalf that I'd only been willing to do for other people. I laid down the hardest bargaining voice I could muster, the hammer of sleep deprivation and work annoyance, and told them over the phone I needed twice the money they were offering. They doubled the pay.

In my second semester of that position, in the early winter of 2005, I experienced my moment of reckoning with the bottle of Odwalla juice in the co-op. That was in some ways the moment that launched this tale, the sinus clog of hopelessness in which I felt I was being taunted by a flyer advertising serenity without health insurance.

The Odwalla moment of this love story holds special meaning for me now, because I can look back and know what my ski-capped then self did not know. My coverage had been wandering around in the world without me. Even as I wrestled with my fear, I had been technically eligible for full health benefits, but no one had told me about it.

It took months for this to become clear. That winter day in my freezing car, I swallowed the last of my juice and talked to Kathy. I recovered from the sinus haze, and the sun warmed the midwestern ground. Looking ahead to a summer without employment, I wrote up multiple proposals for my boss and my boss's boss, describing job configurations and reasons why they might want to employ me through the summer. But I had apparently tapped out that wellspring, and they offered me another contract in the fall. So I applied for a benefits-eligible job on campus teaching journalism and advising the student paper. The position would be grueling but worthwhile for the Frogger résumé-building project. I interviewed and got the job, then broke the happy news to my boss, who understood completely that I needed more security for my family and myself. In the late spring, as the school year was winding down and I was about to switch over to the journalism building, I had finally begun receiving campus mail with some regularity, which had taken several signs and mailboxes in two different mailrooms in the massive College of Engineering complex.

One of those mailers, maybe from Human Resources, happened to list the letter A after my name on the label. With a swelling wave of nausea, I dropped my other tasks and stared at that label. Through years of study and longing, I had memorized the Human Resources benefits categories, and I knew they were coded by letter. I can't explain how, but sweet Jesus, I knew it: No, gods and goddesses of human resources, don't do it. Don't tell me that every moment of stress this past year would disappear into a deep well of meaninglessness and misunderstanding.

I went online and opened the Human Resources benefits spreadsheet. I saw that A was a benefits-eligible job code. Okay, maybe this A next to my name meant something else. I called the Human Resources office in the College of Engineering and was told to call the university's HR. After waiting on hold, clutching the mailer, and trying to breathe, I explained my strange question: "Can you tell me whether I'm an A job code in my current position as lecturer in the College of Engineering?"

The man scrolled and clicked. "Sorry, the computers are freezing up today," he said with a sigh and the sound of clacking keys. "Okay, here we go. Uhhh, yep. Yeah, that's you."

One hundred moments from the previous year flashed before my eyes: waiting on hold to talk to my state healthcare caseworker; faxing in reapplications for my son's coverage; tallying, adding, writing checks; but most of all, the bleak, gray sickness of worry. I wanted to hunt down that worry and stab it, kill whatever had caused each one of those lost moments.

"Can you tell me what campus address you have listed for me?" I asked with the false-calm overenunciation of a woman trying not to lose her shit on someone in customer service who doesn't deserve anonymous abuse.

He read back a general address in the College of Engineering, a third-floor whirlpool of lost mail.

"That would never have reached me," I said.

"Yeah," he said, "it looks like your benefits materials were sent to that address, but they were never returned."

"How could this have happened?" I asked.

He seemed slightly baffled about the emotional and ultimately unknowable nature of my question. He said something like, "Well, you're eligible now; so if you want to sign up, let me know. Is there anything else I can do to help you out today?"

This body—which had been scraping by, unworthy, unsecure, and on the edge—had been important enough that whole year to be insured, to be safe. I hadn't known it. The thin, shining edge of my sickness is that I could feel retroactive self-esteem based on benefits eligibility, that I could also mourn for a year in which hypothetical benefits had gone unused.

Eyes wide, I swiveled my chair to face my boss, who worked in the cubicle opposite me. I tried to explain the grievous error. "That's too bad," he said with a sympathetic wince and a smile. "Sorry about that."

He didn't want to storm the barricades. Never mind—I could summon my own rage. I wanted someone punished, despite the fact that I would soon have benefits through my new job. I didn't know whom to attack. I went down to the College of Engineering's Human Resources office, and the woman there confirmed that the package of benefits materials had probably been misrouted last fall.

Wasn't it a legal requirement, I asked, to have documentation and a signature on file when a benefits-eligible employee refused benefits?

The new HR woman squinted at me. She'd just started the job. Her predecessor didn't have any records of the mailings, she told me, so there was no way she could say for sure what had happened. Certainly there was no human to blame.

Those benefits had been *mine*, I argued. Their retroactive absence from my life was *mine*.

No, said the new HR woman. There was no hole to be documented and filled by the absence of benefits past, no wrong to be righted when dead benefits were found to be missing. They were fringe, decoration, given at the pleasure of the employer and vanishing like daylilies the moment their short life span had passed. Fringe—as in rickrack, tatting, pom-poms, and lace.

I found my car in the parking garage and went home in a daze. My main goal had been to vault myself from benefits wasteland into a "real" position. That was how my friends and I talked over coffee, comparing notes, describing employment, in terms of a *real* job. A real job for a real person. A real person—a real mother—who could afford to pay for health benefits for her real child. Love made the Velveteen Rabbit real; even though time wore out the stuffed animal, its missing stitches and its holes were proof that it was loved. Despite my best intentions and fierce attempts to hunt down security for my family, to love my husband and my child through the actions required to protect them, I'd missed another row of fine print, failed to take into account another slight signal, and spent a year of hypothetical serenity worrying for nothing.

Maslow's pyramid describes an ideal series of progressions from one developmental level to the next, but his system also could be used to explain the outcome of needs denied. In his view, neurosis develops when trauma causes a person to become fixated on a need already met. For example, early experience of hunger—deprivation at the first level of Maslow's pyramid—might lead to lifelong behaviors such as stockpiling food or overeating. Five years after my reckoning with the bottle of Odwalla juice, I can't let go of my healthcare drought or the swirl of days and months and years surrounding the Odwalla moment. I wonder how much of this is neurotic and how much of it is trying to push myself up my own pyramid, driven by level five, the need to understand.

I can look back and feel that moment in the co-op, and I know the horror isn't about my own story. What scares me most about the hopelessness is its uniformity, its commonness, and the way it is parceled out to so many people in our country like rows of Odwalla juice. We open that bottle and drink it and fantasize about a day to come in a land to come, like Canada or Sweden, when we won't have to worry. And then we leave the co-op and we go pick up our children and we raise them with anxiety eating at the edges of our eyes and our smiles, anxiety that is avoidable, inexplicable, and inexcusable.

My new job in the journalism building started in the fall of 2005. I took us off social services, cancelled Skate's catastrophic policy, and enrolled us as a family on one health plan I could almost afford. Even though benefits took a significant bite out of my paycheck each month, it changed how I felt about my entire life. Although I was still slamming the door on the same dented Nissan Sentra each morning and pouring coffee into the same Dollar Store thermos, I felt so ordered and middle-class. We had arrived. We were normal.

When the enrollment package arrived from the benefits administrator, I punched out the laminated card bearing my husband's name and set it carefully on top of his black chain wallet on the kitchen counter. This quiet moment, without any embrace or eye contact, was my movie-scene equivalent of Juliet leaning down over the balcony to Romeo. I found you benefits. Real ones. As much as I can, I have found us a refuge.

To earn the safety, I stepped onto a treadmill so exhausting that I put a blanket and pillow in my Sentra so I could sleep in my car in the university parking lot when I had a free hour. Each morning, I wrote for an hour; then I worked a full day; then I picked Ivan up from daycare, spent the evening with him and Skate, and put Ivan to bed at 8 p.m. Then on most nights, I drove back to work and stayed until midnight or later to wait for the students to finish the next day's edition of the daily campus newspaper.

In my time off I relaxed by running through the gamut of formerly forbidden benefits like optical and women's wellness. I urged Skate to check out the list of chiropractors and take care of his nagging back pain. Or maybe, I suggested, he could finally revisit those teeth and get them fixed up right. He shrugged and reminded me of the last bad dental experience. Or he asked me for the number of a doctor and then never called. Or he went to a few chiropractor appointments, decided it was too much hassle, and quit.

Never mind, I thought. I'll use up enough benefits for both of us. My newest doctor prescribed sprays and steroids for another sinus infection in October 2005. When I returned with another throbbing head, she ran her finger down my chart.

"Hmmmm," she said. "Maybe we should have this checked out."

She wrote me a referral to an otolaryngologist, and I learned how to pronounce that seven-syllable word because "ear, nose, and throat" couldn't convey my joy at getting access to these deep layers of medicine. The otolaryngologist looked up my nose and told me I had chronic sinus inflammation. He stuck his lighted scope up my nostril again and peered upward, twisting my nose around like a vacuum cleaner hose.

"You have a severely deviated septum. Did you have a sharp blow to the face when you were young?" he asked.

I scrolled back through the Rolodex of memories. "I got hit with a basketball once in gym class," I said, remembering the sweat-and-rubber smell of the dirty orange ball.

"Well, it could have been that or a birth defect. In any case, I think we're going to have to do a little surgery," he said. He recommended starting with the bilateral turbinate, spiral-shaped sinus structures on either side of the nose. He would cauterize them back a bit to take down the level of inflammation and maybe the level of pain. Then when I had time for something more involved, we'd do the deviated septum, which would require a more-involved dismantling of my face.

"Great," I said brightly. "If it will help, I'm all for it."

He pulled his lighted scope away from his eye and laughed. "I've rarely had a patient so calm about getting an operation," he said.

"You don't understand," I wanted to tell him. "Cut my face, use your skill, bill my insurance, and I rejoice." The essence of fear is uncertainty. Action, choice, and faith are options that target and pursue a solution, illusory or real, showing the route to sanguine bliss.

As much as it terrified me, the next character-building–insurance-usage adventure was going to have to be my teeth. As I lay looking up at him, my new dentist Dr. K hassled me about the state of my gums and two years' worth of neglect and tartar. I explained that I hadn't had dental insurance.

He nickered softly and said, "If you come in for the cleaning, you save yourself a lot of money down the road."

And I *knew* that. I love saving money. If you compliment me on my skirt, I will say with glee, "I got it for a dollar at Goodwill!" I'm all for preventative maintenance, but thrifty joy is hard to come by at the doctor's office.

But I have avoided seeking help for many minor and maybe kind of major chronic problems because (1) I've already lived with it for ten years anyway; (2) after $975.43 in lab work and $350.08 in co-pays (or $7,480 without insurance), they'll probably tell me it's all in my head; (3) the office visits needed to figure this thing out will require so much time away from work that I'll get fired and lose my insurance; and (4) if it's really serious, it will start to hurt, swell, or bleed, making it easier for them (and cheaper for me) to figure out what's wrong.

I liked Dr. K, though. By the end of that dental visit, he had given me $200 worth of free dental work by polishing out a dark spot on one front tooth and digging out a precavity on a molar. His assistant Cheryl leaned over to tap one of my incisors and asked Dr. K, "Can't we do that one too?"

Dr. K shook his head and flashed his beaten-down yet tragically upbeat smile. Cheryl hunched slighted and stared in a forlorn way at Dr. K's eyes. "You need to get out more, Dr. K," she said. Then she looked down at me, eyes wide with alarm over her paper mask. "He spends all his weekends hanging out on the couch with his dogs."

Dr. K shrugged. "They're great dogs. What can I do?" He fired up the drill again. With a pause from dogs to what they might have replaced, he said, "I don't tell people I was married for twenty-five years. I say a quarter century, because that sounds more impressive." He told a story about the wife, who had thrown a Ginsu knife at him during a fight in the kitchen. "The worst part," he said, "was that she turned around to leave the room. Didn't even watch to see whether the knife had hit me." He shook his head, deadpan, then pulled his fingers out of my mouth so I could laugh and spit.

As he started in on the rotten recesses of the lower left side of my mouth, he squinted with concentration, making wrinkles of crow's-feet near his temples. He *had* been married. He must have felt me staring with a questioning look. He pulled down his mask, leaned back, and popped the overhead light off. "She died of breast cancer," he said.

So of course he was hanging out with his dogs. Dr. K—whom I now loved—refused to make an anonymous saint out of a real woman who happened to have died. He kept her alive as the tempestuous wife. It sounded as if She of the Ginsu Knives would have appreciated it.

At the next dental visit, Dr. K flipped off the interrogation-like lamp above my head, took off his mask, and scrunched his mouth into a grimace. "Well, friend, I thought we were gonna be able to save this one and just do a filling, but we'll have to do a crown."

I hate that mock-happy, fake-royal word, *crown*, like a party hat on a crying kid. "Shit," I said, my heart thrumming. "How much?"

"You've got the fifty-fifty dental plan, so it will run you about five hundred." I looked at him pleadingly, resigned. "I'm sorry," he said.

"We'll see what we can do. But if you don't do this now, it will turn into a root canal, which is way more expensive." *Root canal* at least sounds honest: gripping tentacles and a major cross-continental construction project.

Afterward, I sat in the car with my numb lips and did a little deep breathing. At least this was a devil I knew. I lived in this region of Panic Land; I'd moved in and set up a few end tables and throw rugs. Despite a steady paycheck I had nothing in the bank, and a $500 brake job on my car had gone on the credit card a few days before. My last visit to Dr. K had cost $200, and the sinus issue had so far cost me a $180 co-pay for an MRI. Daycare and rent took me into the negative zone with interest.

I dug for my cell phone in my purse and hit three on my speed dial. "Hey Kath," I said.

"Hey girlfriend," she said. I could hear her kids' voices in the background.

"I'm so broke. I hate this," I laugh-whined.

She groaned sympathetically. "Oh, hon, I know it," she said. Almost as if on the same life schedule, Kathy and I had both finally landed great jobs and health insurance during the same month that summer. After years of WIC and chanting "Progress, Not Perfection," we could both finally flip through our benefits booklets with aplomb and make doctors' appointments just for the hell of it. Kathy had finally gone in for her overdue follow-up mammogram and was waiting for her let's-check-this-it's-probably-nothing appointment next week. Her mom had benign breast cysts. *Nothing to worry about. Nothing to worry about.*

A squeal erupted in the distance on her end.

"Kids fighting?" I asked.

"Freaking out." She laughed again. "Are you okay?"

"Yeah. Thanks for listening. I'm gonna go take a walk and get a coffee before I go back to work," I said.

"Sounds like a plan. Talk later?" Another squeal.

"Cool. Love you. Bye!" We traded the role of cheerleader, urging each other on and watching for signs of that self-castigating voice: "I'm thirty-four. I should have my shit together," was met with a cautionary, "Don't go there. I've got you beat."

In October 2005 I began trolling the job market yet again, this time for a stable job that would allow me to be at home in the evenings with my son. I sent off my packets of syllabi and teaching philosophies, and I had a few interviews. On the trip to visit my parents in Illinois over Christmas, I got to see my sister Nicole, who had moved from Los Angeles to Australia. We left my son with my mom for the day and drove out under gray spitting skies to an outlet mall.

As we drove, we stretched sentences slowly into the silence and listed our worries, bringing each other up to date on our real selves, not the snippets we could reveal in scattered phone conversations a world away. We were united by debt, which scratched its finger-nails on both of our brains. On the way home to Australia, Nicole planned to stop in Los Angeles for a round of checkups and doctors' appointments, including a skin check and a new mouth guard for her jaw disorder. I would realize in the next year that I had many of the same conditions I'd heard Nicole talk about for years, including allergies and the jaw problem. But I had avoided investigating any health problem that wasn't immediately gushing blood or doubling me over in pain. Nicole also needed a test to check out blood in her urine, a mysterious condition she couldn't afford to pursue or investigate in Australia. All of this would have to be paid out of pocket and put on credit.

"Get charity-care applications from each of your doctors' offices in Los Angeles," I said.

She looked at me with brows furrowed. "How the hell did I not know about that?"

We pulled into the mall parking lot under the heavy curved profile of two cooling towers from the nearby nuclear power plant. She wondered if she could stay in Australia and get access to their public health system, which was only available to citizens and residents. Then she turned to me and said she knew I was going to get a good job and would not have to worry.

Someday it will all be easier, we said to each other.

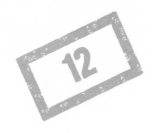

THE PRICE TAG

The Day of Major Dental Reconstruction Appointment Number One arrived in the early winter of 2006. Dr. K worked carefully, switching drill heads to grind my molar into an empty bowl suitable for filling with adhesive to hold my new fake tooth. As the drill vibrated my skull, I closed my eyes and watched for any smidgen of self-pity. No complaining about this pain. It was a privilege. I loved my benefits. *This is easy, you know this is easy, because you know what is after this. This will be fine just as that will be fine.* Kathy's mammogram follow-up at Mt. Carmel Hospital downtown was in an hour, and I was on deck for moral support.

Dr. K took a break to find some adhesive, and I gathered up my dried and stretched-out lips. "Can I take a blreak for a thecond? I need to call a thriend and tell her I'll be late," I said. I reached into my bag for my cell phone, left Kathy a message on her voice mail, and settled back into the chair.

I paused. "She's having a breast biopsy," I said.

"What does she have?" Dr. K asked. "Is it fibrocystic disease? Is it intraductal papilloma?"

"I don't think they know yet," I said.

At the end of the visit, he scrawled a note on my chart and told me to hand it to the cashier. He'd knocked $100 off my bill.

The top level of the hospital garage, submerged in fog and midwestern gray, felt like a barge floating on the North Sea. I parked and jogged to the clinic entrance. Even today, I remember that moment: crossing the gray cement, with two possibilities of malignant or benign, the breathless and muffled stopped time of not knowing, as denial fell away and I admitted to myself that there were two options.

I pulled the door open to the waiting room. Kathy looked up, smiling her calm, gentle smile; her parents stood to grab my hands and hug me. Kathy looked a bit peaked with a feverish flush, a little edgy, a little red around the eyes. Kathy's mom was bright and chatty, her dad a bit subdued. I felt my way gently into the mood. I guessed that mindless chatter might be appropriate to fill the minutes while Kathy waited to be called back to the exam room.

"I just came from the dentist. Five hundred dollars for a crown!" I said.

Kathy pulled her cheek to tap at a back tooth. "I've had a temporary crown on there for six months," she said. "I keep pushing at it, trying to see if it hurts."

Her dad smiled. "If it hurts, maybe you shouldn't push at it anymore," he said. We laughed at the dadness of his response.

Kathy said, "I want to see how much it hurts. If it's going to need a root canal anyway, I'm not going to pay for the crown."

The economic banter was light, distracting, a fuzz of peroxide in an open wound, like cutting in order to clean. And my chest pinched slightly as I saw both her and myself on an average day: driving around Columbus in the overcast gloom, rushing to pick up children, rushing between work and appointments, Kathy working to become a hospital chaplain, filling out permission slips for school trips, packing lunches, and finding time to stop to buy soy milk and toilet paper.

A nurse with a manila folder opened a door and called, "Kathy," with an upward inflection, as if the name were also a question. Which it was.

The waiting room was decorated in comforting greens with maybe a homey touch of ruffled floral curtains, much nicer than an eighties institutional gray. Kathy's mom twittered and nodded, asking about my life. She told me about a Catholic antiwar conference she'd been to in Washington DC. I obliged the need for distraction, feeding the tangent. We talked about Anne Lamott, an author who spoke at the conference and scandalized the Catholics with her honesty. We waited, glancing out the windows at the unmoving gray, knowing that Kathy was being poked in there, that cells were being removed, and that those cells knew more than we did.

"I couldn't believe Annie said the ef word," said Kathy's mom, laughing into her hand. Lamott, a featured speaker at the conference, had gotten riled up about the issue of abortion.

I listed my favorite Anne Lamott books and promised to lend her one. She asked if I'd read the Catholic contemplative Thomas Merton, then told me the conference ended with the participants standing all in a circle. They grasped hands and then turned outward, extending their palms as they envisioned compassion and love flowing to those who needed it, to the men, women, and children of Iraq.

How long had we been waiting? It felt too long. I glanced at my watch—twenty minutes or so—then grasped for another topic. I asked about Kathy's siblings, and Kathy's mom glanced toward the reception desk, mouth half open in thought.

"You know, Kathy had the lump two years ago," she said. That information sat between the three of us, and queasiness bloomed in my stomach. Yes. I remembered now, hearing about the mammogram two years ago. The same lump that had been declared "nothing: let's just keep an eye on it." But now the duration, the length of Kathy's relationship with this lump, seemed nauseating. As Kathy's mom told more of the story, she patted the air in a downward circular motion to emphasize passage of time, a gentle gesture of Kathy's that I loved. "They said then that it seemed like a fibroid," Kathy's mom said.

We paused again. Her mom and dad glanced at each other, and his watery eyes searched hers. She looked back at me.

"Then last year, she didn't have the money or insurance for a mammogram, so she decided to wait."

Last year was the finalization of Kathy's divorce, of sleeping with three beds crammed into one small basement room of her parents' house. She finished her certification classes and got her first shifts as a part-time hospital chaplain, overnight and on call with a beeper. She flew and drove back and forth between Ohio and Minnesota to sort out a real estate dispute with her former husband.

So she decided to wait. And sitting there, none of us judged her for that. We said nothing, but I could feel it. It was a fact, as solid as her temporary crown, as edgeless as the gray outside.

Minutes later, the door opened and Kathy emerged. We probably all stood and looked at her intently, too expectantly. She grabbed her coat. Then, tipping off kilter, she wobbled on her feet. "They didn't even do a biopsy today. This was just a 'get to know you.'" She was coasting down from an adrenaline high, tamped down by regret. She wanted the lump out of her.

"It's probably filled with fluid. That's why it looks solid on the mammogram. That's what happened with mine," her mom said. We knew this: her mom had had a benign "nothing," but her grandmother had died of breast cancer.

We drove to a local Irish pub to drink beer and eat nachos, fried potato pancakes, and stuffed potato wedges. We talked about a friend who had committed suicide a few days before. It had been a particularly rough week.

Three days later, I flew to Georgia for a job interview, a high-stakes tryout for a tenure-track college teaching job. I called Kathy from the airport, twirling the stirrer of my Starbucks coffee as she joked with me about how I'd blow their minds, how I didn't need to worry, how the hard part of getting in the door was done.

And she was scheduled for the biopsy on the same day as my interview. We both stood on some kind of precipice, hoping for rescue, but I felt as though all I had to say were stupid platitudes.

"It's going to be nothing. Then when I get back, I'll take you out for a celebratory beer or three," I said.

"And then you'll get the job in Georgia, and you'll leave me!" she laugh-cried.

"I'll always be around to bother you," I said. "You'll never get rid of me."

Throughout my job interview the next day—the presentations, the discussion of my curriculum vitae, and my presentation of a Stepford-candidate version of myself—I kept a grip on my cell phone. Somehow waiting for Kathy's news put my small drama in perspective and even kept me calm. This is just a job. It's not cancer. Well, that's not cancer either. Nothing is cancer.

But it was.

Friday morning, another Starbucks call in an airport, and . . . oh.

Oh, Kathy. No.

And then we were in it, submerged in that rushing of cancer time that picks you up like a torrent, altering everything in its image. I sat down and cried, careful to keep my face away from the mouthpiece so I wouldn't betray my helplessness with breathing and snuffling.

"Oh, Kath."

"It's stage one," she said. "That's the best kind."

"Hey, the good kind of cancer!" I joked. Then I started to cry but stopped myself. "How soon did they know? How long did you have to wait?"

"I thought they were going to aspirate this fluid-filled thing. The doctor gave me a local anesthetic and went in to try to get at it, said she'd try to take it out right there. Then she kept tugging at it, said it wasn't supposed to be connected to the tissue around it, wasn't supposed to be hard . . ."

"Fuck." I bit my lip to keep the coffee in my stomach, saw black splotches. I did not want to imagine the probe in her flesh encountering anything solid. Her flesh.

"I knew. They didn't tell me exactly right then, but I could see it on the doctor's face. She just got really quiet." Kathy paused, took a breath, told me a bit more about the rush toward surgery that had exploded around her. All of a sudden she had to decide by Monday whether to do breast reconstruction. She'd be in the hospital in less than a week for the mastectomy.

"So . . . well, that's the cancer. How did the interview go?" she asked brightly.

I stared at the lip of my white Starbucks paper cup, a clinical curl like the edge of a hospital gown. Like in the waiting room last week, I knew my job now was to provide distraction, to sew us both to normal life. "It was great. I loved it—it's beautiful here. Green—I flew out of Dayton in a snowstorm and landed in sun. I think I did really well," I said. "And the people are wonderful." I chattered and refelt the joy of the interview as I recounted the details. We were not cancer and cancer's friend. We were moms, career women, women with mistakes behind us and joy ahead.

A few hours later, I touched down into gray Ohio and drove to Kathy's house. I hugged her, and she didn't feel like cancer. And I had a strange disbelief, the illusion that I'd made it up and could unthink it somehow.

We spent the afternoon together, running errands, buying milk, and laughing as Kathy's train of thought derailed. This was something concrete I could offer—wicked humor, tangential jokes, distraction. We went for an organic lunch at a local vegetarian restaurant called Benevolence. We saw the man who'd performed my wedding ceremony, a minister and feng shui consultant.

Kathy ate a salad, and we talked about the pointlessness and sadness of trying to be organic and poison free now with massive chemo looming. I tried to imagine what I would say if I were Kathy—if I were gentle and focused, a born listener and the asker of soulful, thoughtful questions. But all I had to offer was my swearing, joke-cracking self, veering at unexpected moments into tears she didn't need.

We wheeled a shopping cart through Target and laughed about how you could get lost here, how it was the mom's version of a bubble bath. "Maybe I should get my nails done," she said. She turned the cart into the aisle of lotions and shampoos, near the pharmacy. "God, I have to think about what I'll need in the house to make me feel better after the surgery." The bare bones necessities: toilet paper, Kleenex. Painkillers and fluid drainage and gauze.

She grabbed a bottle of scented body lotion and held it over the open mouth of the cart, stopping in midair. We looked at the plastic bottle. Without saying anything, it was clear to both of us that this was some kind of new desperation where neither of us had been, something that lotion could not fix.

She wobbled again. "You better push the cart," she said.

Two days later, we gathered in a living room, five women friends, to drink wine and talk about boobs, to ask Kathy questions about her upcoming surgery and the biopsy. She answered with details about the procedure and accidentally used the word *mammogram* every time she meant *mastectomy*. No one corrected her.

"Do you want to see?" she asked, suddenly shy. "This is their last appearance." She grabbed the hem of her shirt and then hesitated.

I yanked up my shirt. "Look, you can see mine," I said. "I'll go first." I peeled back the lower edge of my bra, and my skin met the cool air. "See what breast-feeding has done to me? It's like sand in a Ziploc bag." I jiggled the skin to make my small, flat boob quiver.

Using my boobs every day for feeding had transformed them into something about as erotic as the kitchen sink. The girls howled and laughed.

"Mine's the same way," Kathy said. "And what am I supposed to do, get the other breast reconstructed so it's saggy to match my left one?"

Then she raised her shirt, and we sighed and argued with her, murmured compliments in the way that women always secretly admire each others' bodies. The breast was beautiful, even with the green and yellow biopsy bruise: small and rounded, with a large mauve pink nipple. "Somehow, the part about losing the nipple is the scariest," she said, looking down at it.

"It's like the eyes on a face," I said, and we laughed.

We drank more wine, and the fire blurred orange. We prayed that the cancer had not gone into the lymph nodes. We talked about a 40 percent chance of recurrence, which Tamoxifen could reduce. One of the women was into Reiki, a hands-on healing thing with energy, and she told us to stand around Kathy and put our hands around her shoulders.

Part of me wanted to roll my eyes, to flinch and say, "This is so hokey," I lectured myself to stand up straight, to let go of any illusions that I was in control here. Our job is to do anything, anything that might help.

We laughed and danced, then settled back down to eat brownies and drink more wine.

"I feel like I owe my boob an apology," Kathy said later. She pulled at the neckline of her shirt, laughing, and said down into the fabric, "I'm sorry for apologizing for you. I'm sorry for the push-up bras and for ignoring you."

Kathy repeated the story of this lump to try to make sense of it. Two years ago, she said, the doctors told her the lump was a fibroadenoma, a kind of tissue that does not change into cancer.

They were wrong. That meant the lump had been some form of cancer or precancer for two years. She scheduled a mammogram when she felt it getting bigger.

"And so," she asked, looking up with a clear-eyed, searching question, "what does it mean about me? That I'm getting cancer because somehow I was too stressed out? Because I didn't take good enough care of myself?"

Down the rabbit hole we went with her, into the agony of wondering what might have been if she'd had the lump checked sooner. We wouldn't let her go there alone, and it was our job to haul her out of there. We hardly ever saw this side of Kathy, who is so conscious to stay positive, so willing and able to pull each of us out when we get to the brink in our own lives.

It's stage one, we argued, how much sooner could it be? She had been busy getting a divorce and raising two kids. You are good enough, we said, and you did what you could. We talked over, through, and around, because there was no use saying that we were pushing back against an extra helping of horror and fear. It was not laziness or lack of self-care. The horror was lack of money, energy, attention, and days on the calendar.

It was late, and I had to get home to feed the baby with my wilting boobs. I grabbed my car keys and my jacket, then hugged Kathy and the others. My face, bathed in cool night air, felt hot from the fire and the wine. The next day was my thirty-fifth birthday and the Tibetan New Year; the confluence might have seemed magical and auspicious once. But my birthday faded into an earlier life, when the childlike notion of each year was a discrete and separate project and adventure. I prayed as I drove through the dark night, which was shot with white spots of light. I imagined that I was high up on elevated tracks, that my hope and positive feelings could ensure somehow that the cancer was not in the lymph nodes.

This tragedy did not feel like a Lifetime movie script, and the

evening of wine and women and laughter was not a redemptive circling of the wagons that made us all feel at peace. Instead, we were
children, little girls, driven down to the very last things we had in our
bags of tricks. With a child's clinging to never-never land, I said in
my quiet, cold car, "It didn't have to be this way." Since I was alone,
I could surrender to what we fought against all night. I pounded the
steering wheel and started to scream in my car at the universe, at
the cold, at the mammogram that cost $125 too much. I pulled over
out of traffic and wiped my wet face. If there was serenity there, it
was the tragic serenity of the sentenced, those who cross beyond
rage or depression, those who will do anything to make this right
and have lost themselves in the fire of that need.

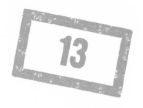

FOLLOWING UP

I accepted a full-time teaching job in Georgia, and in summer of 2006 Skate and I packed boxes and put our house up for sale. I was leaping into a new and challenging job with security and the first comprehensive benefits package of my life at age thirty-five. In asking Skate to leave Ohio, I ripped him away from his home ground, the place where he'd lived his whole life. I bought guidebooks of coastal Georgia to try to make our move seem like a vacation. I kept packing, driven to push toward security, even if it tore apart my marriage in the process.

The month before we left town, Ivan and I were rear-ended at an intersection near our home. In the seconds before the car behind us collided with our bumper, I had reached around to hand Ivan a Fruit Roll-Up, so the impact gave me whiplash and a wrenched right shoulder. I had never been to a bone cracker but had to do something; my hands were numb on the computer keyboard. Like every other mover toward health, I learned about preventative care through an emergency.

The chiropractor showed me a full-body x-ray of myself and pointed out with his pen on the film how my hips were cockeyed from holding Ivan on one side. "All mothers get this," he said. "And we can fix it." He showed me a side view of my head and told me that I was missing a curve in my neck. "This is called military neck. You must have fantastic headaches," he said. Then he grabbed my skull and pointed at the places where he guessed I had pain. The vertebrae unfolded like flowers, and I was stunned at the small pressure of fingertips and their power to change reality.

My last round of benefits statements from my Ohio insurance plan detailed a range of services including massages, ultrasound treatments for the pain, exercise consultation, and strength build-ing. The idea of a stranger's hands on me for a massage would have terrified me if I hadn't been in such pain. Ami and Kathy had given me a gift certificate for a massage at my wedding shower, and I had never used it. The hot pain radiating from my neck forced me into the attic studio at the chiropractor's office, where floaty dolphin music bubbled in the background. I lay on the clean sheet and studied an anatomy poster tacked to the wall. I held my breath as the massage therapist's hands contacted my skin and his fingers pushed into muscles that jumped and relaxed.

Two weeks before we left for Georgia, I gave my son a disposable camera to take pictures of his people and places in Columbus. His skewed two-year-old framing captured a diagonal shot of a bald Kathy, nearing the end of chemotherapy, laughing with sweet glee and blocking her eyes from the glare of Ivan's flash. We had been counting down all spring to the day of Kathy's final round of chemo. We wanted to have a chemo party before I left, but her exhaustion overlapped my cardboard boxes, as the final chemo came just days before the moving truck would pull away.

Skate and I unpacked in Georgia and braved the heat. That fall of 2006, I navigated paperwork and passwords on a southern campus draped in Spanish moss. I carefully covered my tattoos, lusted after coffee shops, and researched the nearest bookstores as I acclimated to the rural south. In October, just after our benefits cards finally arrived in the mail, my husband, son, and I went up to New York

City for the wedding of my friend Brooke to her girlfriend Peg. They
had been together for five years and had been trying to have a child
by in vitro fertilization. Credit card debt accrued, and relief finally
came when Brooke got a job with a city antidiscrimination legal
office with benefits for domestic partners. After a trip to Canada for
a legal wedding, they had organized a second ceremony and party
for friends; we soaked in the rich coffee, smells of food, and traffic of
Brooklyn. I was happy to see the kisses and embraces between Peg
and Brooke, but I hardened my heart against the strains of sweet
dance music and the lyrics' promises of safety ever after.

Pollen fell from the pine trees of southeast Georgia and coated the
car in a gummy yellow haze. In the afternoon light, the car windshield
glittered like gold. Pollen accumulated in a scrim along the gut-
ters, washed into bright high-water lines by the rain. It even drifted,
forming a yellow dusty slope in the concrete gap of two adjoining
buildings on campus. The fecundity of spring in the country of Lob-
lolly Pine—oak and maple, magenta and fuchsia flowering azalea
bushes, cotton, and wiregrass—forced me from Sudafed to the shelf
of over-the-counter medicine that promised to dry out one's sinuses
like beef jerky. Another sinus infection and the dumb-headed allergy
clog impeded my ability to think. So when a colleague mentioned
her allergist in passing conversation, I shyly approached her. How
did you get one of those?

With the allergist's name and number, I thumbed through my
health benefits plan, which included chiropractic, partial reimburse-
ment for massage and acupuncture, and other wildly unimaginable,
cheap, and noninvasive care options. How hilarious, adult, and sane.
How Canadian. I had heard about this thing called preventative medicine, but I had been too busy visiting emergency rooms over the last
twenty years to look into it.

At the allergist's office, I took off my shirt and lay face down on the exam table. A nurse drew a grid in Magic Marker on my back. She carried in a metal tray with a crowd of tiny glass vials, each containing an essence of a common allergen. She pricked my skin with the needles, one by one, then told me to relax for fifteen minutes. My skin itched as it etched a visible map, red circles and bumps that rose in a mathematically readable response, a page of me describing what did not agree with my system.

I lay on the crinkly paper sheet, remembering a childhood and early adulthood of phlegm. Of coughing in classrooms and church, of forcing down the cough and then getting up with red-faced effort and going out into the hall for a coughing fit so hard it made me sweat and see black spots. Of the raw-throated feeling of knowing that each cough made the next one more likely. Of hacking late at night and sucking on Sucrets, of Chloraseptic spray, of reading stories in the bathroom with Mom at 2 a.m. as steam rose from a running hot shower so I could breathe. Of sleeping angled up on pillows so the phlegm would drain down my throat instead of causing the cough, of my mom buying hypoallergenic blankets, of my parents smoking. Of the gradually increasing dependence on Sudafed to get through days, weeks, months, and years. Of the Husten—the coughs in my German family—which my mom's relatives assume will develop in each of them because we have weak lungs or because we come from a coal-mining area in the northwest of that country.

The nurse reappeared with the doctor. She touched some device I couldn't see to the skin on my back and measured each wheal, reading its size and height to the doctor in a series of paired numbers he wrote in rows on his clipboard. They both disappeared, but she came back with a long list of substances, mostly plants, that my body is allergic to: pine, saw palmetto, grasses, mites, dogs and cats. It was my portrait in reference to the outside world. I got dressed.

The doctor returned and said he wanted to explain my results. He touched my face, looked in my eyes with a stillness that I found disconcerting. He studied my eyes with calm observation, taking me in. Seeing me. I looked away to break eye contact, glancing at a corner of the exam room. I had not been looked at that way in a long time. There was such clinical care in his fingertips as he touched my face that I wanted to cry.

"Some puffiness in the face, discharge in the eyes," he said. He used a lit scope to peer up into my nose. "Ahh-hmmm. Your sinuses are inflamed." He pressed the skin under my cheekbone. "Does this hurt?" he asked. I flinched.

"Open your mouth," he said. His fingers moved lightly at the underside of my jawbone, touching lymph nodes and edging back toward my ears. I moved my jaw. "Can you open it any wider?" he asked. The jaw had a trick to it; I had to angle it partway open, then kind of shift it to the side to get it to open wide, like a busted car door. I managed it in a rough two-step sliding process. "Again," he said. I tried to do the open-shift-open a bit faster.

"Do you have jaw pain?" he asked.

I sighed. "Yeah. My face, my teeth, all of it."

He crossed his arms and looked at me. "I think you have TMJ," he said, and then explained the condition called temporomandibular joint complex disorder. He glanced down at my chart, then up at me, clear-eyed and calm with maybe a bit of compassion or sadness there, too. "TMJ is linked to depression, neck pain, tooth pain, and sinus trouble. You're not getting the sleep you need because you're probably breathing through your mouth at night, aggravating the jaw. You may have been sleep deprived for years, and all that in addition to the chronic pain is a lot to bear."

My TMJ remembers the shred and jar of both whiplash car accidents, the overforced pry of rough and misguided root canals, and the openmouthed breathing of thousands of nights around stuffed sinuses. Under stress and worry, the jaw muscles clench like fists. Pushed beyond their limits, the muscles constrict blood flow, squeeze nerves, inflame sinuses, impede pain messages, and pop their own joints out of socket. Misaligned joints pulverize their own cartilage, shatter the teeth they are meant to guide, and spread muscle injury and bone misalignment as far as the neck, spine, and shoulders. Though I massage my jaw to relax it, though I ice it and baby it and buffer it each night with a mouth guard, it has become a new machine marked by its experience. Now it will tighten until my heart stops beating.

Our ancestors' jaw power cracked seed and bone for survival, and the calories won by the mandible and molars powered our evolution. The temporomandibular joint complex beneath each of your ears orchestrates your sip, smile, and sing as it coordinates both up-and-down and side-to-side motion. Like any partnership, the paired joints must work fluidly, each bearing half the burden. Like any marriage, tension and pain untreated can amplify, spreading wounds and dislocations until the phantoms of pain pervade and the original cause is almost impossible to discern.

The summer of 2007, after my first year in Georgia, meant a trip back to Ohio for a teacher-training institute at Ohio State University. I noticed myself looking forward to leaving home. The first years of our marriage showed the strains of two people pulling in opposite directions. I failed to come up with any intelligent alternative and, when I was exhausted with the struggle, simply withdrew. An explosive conversation with car keys already in hand led me to say what I wanted: to end it.

But then we tried one more year, which was both hopeful and difficult. In May and June of 2008, I left Georgia again with my son to tour the Midwest on a low-budget book tour. The pull of the highway and the calm that came with leaving let me know that the marriage was coming apart, once and for all, despite my will and best intentions. The relief of seeing old friends up north also meant time in the

car facing the rolling blacktop, time to think. I called it my Midwest
meditation retreat. I fell into the rhythm of switching CDs, gassing
up, and finding exits as I mulled over the past year.

I saw my old punk-rock friend Steve with his new wife and short
haircut. I reconnected with my old friend Arwen, whom I had lost
touch with but who strangely enough knew Kathy's sister Kristen in
Minneapolis. Kristen had passed along a thick packet of photos and
a letter from me, and our e-mails led to a visit. Arwen welcomed me
with the same bright eyes and hugged me with lithe dancer's arms.
She invited me into her home, blocks away from where we'd first
worked together at the coffee shop. We stepped across a tumble of
shoes in the entryway, Arwen's and her partner's and their young
daughter's. Arwen and I sat in a sunlit window seat in a house she
owned, and we talked about the struggle of planning, of desire.

After a reading in Chicago, I left my son with my parents in Illinois and headed east to Ohio for a few more events, with time to
see Kathy in between. She gave me directions to her new house in
Bexley, Ohio, one of the wealthiest suburbs of Columbus. She and
her kids had just moved in with her boyfriend, David. I found their
house by looking for her old, red London-style mailbox, which she'd
hung on the green siding of the Bexley house.

Kathy sat on the back porch in the sun and motioned for me to
pull up a chair. She turned gingerly, favoring her middle and the
fresh hysterectomy scar. The surgery was a common preventative
measure for women who'd survived her kind of cancer. She turned
her freckled face up to the blue sky to catch the warmth of the sun.
"I'm sick of the surgeries," she said quietly. "This had better be the
last one."

David came out to the porch and set a few drinks on the glass
tabletop, and they chatted about weekend plans and picking up the
kids. She turned to me. "You seem like you're doing really good,"
she said, looking at me with her calm eyes.

"I am," I said. Maybe it was being able to hold a copy of my first book, the three-pound heft of physical validation. Or maybe it was the friends I'd visited in Minneapolis, Chicago, and Ohio, people who knew me as far back as twenty years ago. In each city, at each dinner over spinach pie or stir-fry or steak, I caught in my friends' eyes glimpses of myself in earlier times—a scrapbook, a yardstick, and a reminder. I felt at those dinners and coffees as if I were being invested with the gossamer cutouts of my laughing self at twenty, twenty-five, thirty, the outlines of a scrappy girl not so much ruled by fear, a woman who believed in more than white-knuckling it through the weeks.

I have been good at dealing with chronic pain. When chronic pain stops, it is like background noise silenced: the stunning space rushes at you like a full, blank sky under a flat horizon. There was no cartilage left to buffer my six-year marriage and ten-year relationship. It was bone on bone, and I hadn't realized that temporary ailments can become permanent, can change the shape of the body itself. One version of my story is that good healthcare—appointments, cleanings, long-delayed annual exams, preventative care—swept clean a space of worry in which I could imagine other needs and wants. I believe in Maslow's pyramid, that the brain and body, cared for and calmed, begin to unfold and assess, to measure the trek further upward.

I picked up Ivan at my parents' house in Illinois and drove back down to Georgia, knowing as I did that the second attempt to end my marriage was already internally launched. To steer away from panic, I focused on the simple list of things I could do to reduce pain in my life. I kept all my doctors' appointments and got referrals to specialists. One thing at a time.

The jaw doctor clipped my x-rays to a light box and tapped the ghostly image of my molars with his pen. "This is classic late-stage TMJ," he said. "You have strong teeth. They've just been crushed."

I stared at my x-ray, the filled and false molars with cloudy hearts. I'd seen the same picture so many times in dentists' offices, but the teeth looked sad today, misunderstood. I felt old, mortal—that film was a version of my autobiography, written in two rows of battered dentin and enamel. The jaw doctor peered again at the x-ray. "How's your hearing?"

"Ringing. And hearing my students—I've had trouble," I said. "I thought it was a stuffy head." I had even, out of annoyance, begun to put my hand up to my ear in the classroom, and had started telling students I had hearing problems—not because I really did, of course, but just to make them talk louder.

The doctor reached toward his desk to grab a model of the jaw joint. Pink strands of plastic muscle wrapped around the skinless half face like ribbons on a birthday present. The doctor tapped near the ear to show me how the eustachian tubes ran near the jaw joint. "The muscles swell and press on the auditory nerves," he said. "We'll put you on a soft diet and see whether there's been permanent nerve damage. Given the degree of pain you're in and the condition of the joint, I think the best thing to consider might be surgery."

He made a plaster impression of my top row of teeth, and his assistant fit a strip of plastic along the cast to make me a mouth guard, which I was to wear every night and basically any other time I kept my mouth shut for an extended period of time. I paid them $800 for the mouth guard. Within two days of wearing it, I felt like someone had given me a new skull or inflated the old one with champagne. I learned the outline of the pain by its absence. A week later, the dog ate the mouth guard, and I wrote an $800 check for a second one.

Pain can end. In that month of July, amid Georgia heat and reckoning with x-rays and damage, my marriage was done. By the time the second mouth guard was shaped in plastic and pressed into the plaster mold of my bite impression, I was a single mom. My husband left for Ohio with a vanload of his stuff. I worried about his benefits, promised him I would keep him on my plan until the divorce was final.

Although it was difficult to connect by phone with my sister Nicole that fall, we exchanged bits and pieces of news about her job and my divorce proceedings in instant messages and e-mails.

"The job is up in the air," she said with a sigh, during one of my late nights and her workdays. I struggled to picture her face—her voice so close, still twinged with nasal Chicago South Side but vowels also flattened a bit by three years of Australian twang. "I have to stay awhile longer if I want to get a shot at residency, but think about it. I could always come back here for healthcare. If anything were to ever happen," she said.

We both paused, imagining wordlessly the fears of future cancer and other ailments, the shadow of financial chaos. And that unexpected comfort to cushion her life, the home base of Australian healthcare. She would later learn that Australian healthcare had its own complications and restrictions, but we were both so enamored of the fantasy that we each saw it as a good project to devote a few years of her life to.

"Totally," I said. "You can't pass that up."

When she arrived back in Los Angeles that December, it was partly to put her remaining furniture in storage and tie up a few loose ends. Before selling her old desktop computer, she needed to take out the hard drive. When she reached in to grab it, she sliced open her finger on a loose edge of metal.

When she told me the story later, we could barely hear each other through the howling laughter. "I can't believe I'm laughing at this," I said. "I'm evil."

"I'm telling you this because I knew you would appreciate it," she said. "I wrapped my bleeding hand in a pair of pants. I'm bleeding all over the place, through the pants, and I'm on my laptop looking for directions to the nearest urgent care places, because I don't remember anything about LA. And then I'm calling to see who can offer me the best deal. Blood all over the place and I'm swearing and Googling."

December in southeast Georgia bathed the air in sunlight and a cool, pine-scented breeze. A native midwesterner of the cornfield variety, I noticed the pine smell every time I got out of the car at the grocery store; it was more sandy and subtle than evergreen or Christmas tree. At home I hung up a few strands of Christmas lights and put up the fake tree, but my son was with his father and would wake up Christmas Day to the sight of his grandmother's decorated tree in Ohio. To get my son back to Georgia and to traverse the grid of holidays on the calendar, I had a problem to solve: Georgia to Ohio to my parents in Illinois to Georgia, a Bermuda Triangle of Christmas road trips. More important than the holiday was the moment I got my son into my arms, felt his soft skin and smelled his boy-rainwater smell, buckled him into his car seat.

I called Kathy. "What are you doing Christmas Eve?" I asked. "This might be totally uncool to ask, but I need a place to crash in Columbus."

"That's so awesome," she said, laughing. "Of course you can stay. I love this. It's like *Friends*. I love that I am the person you call to stay with on Christmas."

I laid facedown between Laura's legs and uttered a prayer of stunned gratitude that my insurance covered massage therapy for cases of TMJ. Laura sat on a stool and leaned toward me, pressing the heels of her palms into the tops of my shoulders.

"You better wear that mouth guard the whole time you're driving up to Ohio next week, girl," said Laura.

"I know, I know," I said. "I will."

Pain hardened in a necklace of cinnamon red hots from my jaw down the tops of my shoulders with muscles layered around these cores of poison. Behind closed eyes, I was inside that lava shell of pain, pressing outward to dimly sense the tree trunks of my limbs and head. Laura's fingertips worked toward the heat. I focused into the pain and then gave up, moaning and swearing.

"God. Owwwwwww. Ouch."

"Do you want me to stop?"

"No," I said. "It's good. I know it's a good thing."

Her fingertips moved lightly to touch the old scar on the top of my right shoulder. "What is this from?" she asked.

"Hemangioma," I said. "A strawberry birthmark. It was open, or something like that, when I was born, and they had to cut it out."

She touched into the scar. "And the pain is worse right underneath here, right?" She pushed steadily into the scar, into the spot that made me fear back rubs.

"Dammit!" I said. "Sorry." I began to sweat.

"This might be scar tissue," she said, pulling gently at the muscles beneath. She dug with her thumbs into the area beneath the scar. I started to cry and bit my lip. "This is a trigger point. It could be pulling everything out of whack." She worked at it a bit more then laid heated rocks on the shoulder to calm it.

When she turned me over to work on my jaw, tiny cavities and fissures seemed to pop inside my skull and face. I heard a crackle in my right ear and felt a whoosh of air in the sinus cavity below my left eye. My scalp expanded. Vertebrae in my neck separated audibly with a series of clicks. A huge heat seemed to bloom under my scalp.

"Oh my God," I said. "Oh God. I . . . The inside of my head is all coming apart."

"Those are your sinuses and your muscles, honey. It's all con-nected," she said, and laughed. She stopped, looking down. "Yep. Your face looks different now."

After she finished, I shrugged on my shirt and caught a look in the mirror. It was me, of course, but my cheekbones angled outward and my jaw had dropped. The very shape of whom I knew as myself was changed in one hour by someone's hands, by someone who knew what to touch and what to release.

I picked at a platter of Christmas cookies. "I'm eating all the chocolate ones," I called to Kathy. "I guess I better eat dinner first."

Kathy peered into her refrigerator. "I have beer. A little hummus from the staff Christmas party. Do you want some of that?"

I ladled two paper bowls of potato-leek soup from the Crock-Pot near the sink. I passed one to my new boyfriend, sitting at the counter, who accompanied me on this trek. He smiled as Kathy and I attempted to catch up in shorthand.

She glanced at Cliff, raised her eyebrows at me, and smiled. I left the kitchen to run upstairs for a sweater, glad to hear Cliff chatting with Kathy in a way that provoked laughter, her high sounds of delight and his infectious baritone infused with mock outrage, telling a story at his own expense about some road trip disaster.

I came back downstairs, and Kathy turned to me. "Kristen's coming over," she said. "And I think Laura and her baby. We're having a party, and I didn't even plan one!" Kathy's boyfriend David was working, flying holiday travelers in the cloudy sky above us on Christmas Eve. Her kids were with her ex-husband and his new wife.

"Look at your hair!" I said. I rubbed my fingers in it and then wrapped my arms around her as she stood in front of the open refrigerator. Since the chemo, her hair was soft, dark, and curly, the longest I'd ever seen it.

She showed Cliff and me up to her daughter's room, an explosion of pink and glitter. I lay down on the bed and touched the dresser next to me. I recognized its shape, despite the bright red paint and white stars and stickers. I had received the bureau somehow in an

East Coast breakup with my college boyfriend fifteen years before, when it was painted white. It had moved with me to Chicago, then to Columbus, where I painted it dark red and used it to hold my son's baby clothes. When I moved to Georgia, the dresser found a home with Kathy. It seemed rejuvenated, happy in its new incarnation.

After the introductions and the party and laughter, before going to sleep, I slipped downstairs and curled up on the leather couch under an afghan to talk with Kathy in shorthand about the single-mother worries, fears, and hurdles crossed. About kids and boyfriends and merged households, about money and health as temporary and borrowed. I leaned my neck against the leather armrest as we talked, pressing into sore neck muscles and massaging my jaw. I squinted to make the colored lights on the Christmas tree merge into blurred balls of orange, red, and blue.

The next morning, I woke up and dressed in a jangle of nerves in the quiet house, eager and nervous to pick up my son from his father's house. I turned the key, and a slight riffle of snow furled from the windshield. I put on the John Cougar Mellencamp CD Cliff had bought the day before and turned it up loud, listening in a crackle through my low-budget speakers. I prayed for a calm exchange. Then I found left and right turns, and merged onto the Columbus outer belt. The scatter of silver snow caught pale light through heavy clouds, twinkling like snow-globe snow.

"Merry Christmas," I said in my head to the few cars I passed on the eight-lane highway. Who would be driving at 8 a.m. on Christmas morning? I knew that in each of those cold cars there was a story that overlapped with mine.

Here I am, exhausted and beyond nervous, going into yet another of those situations in which I did not expect to ever find myself. Planless despite the best of intentions, jumping once again and making stability in midflight, grounding myself with reference to what has already passed, telling myself this is easy because of whatever else I have lived through. I am on the highway, and these people who happen to be on the highway on Christmas morning, these are my people. Let us all find shelter and then something beyond.

IN THE CLASS IN AMERICA SERIES

Cover Me
A Health Insurance Memoir
Sonya Huber

To order or obtain more information on these or other University of
Nebraska Press titles, visit www.nebraskapress.unl.edu.